Strength and Physique

High Tension Exercises for Muscular Growth

By James Chan

Strength and Physique

High Tension Exercises for Muscular Growth

By James Chan

Published 2012

Manufactured in the United States of America.

Dedication

I dedicate this book to my lovely wife. I would not have been able to write this book or my previous books had it not been for her support. Had I not met my wife, I would have been lying in a proverbial ditch. She has made me the best version of me.

I also dedicate this book to my father, who was my model of strength.

About the Author

James Chan is a police officer for the University of California. During his career, James has served as a police detective and as a defensive tactics instructor. A former NSCA certified personal trainer, James has written articles for Bodybuilding.com, T-Nation and Planet Muscle magazine.

To tap into his insights on strength training and bodybuilding, visit his blog at:

www.strengthandphysique.blogspot.com

TABLE OF CONTENTS

INTRODUCTION

Want to know the secret to ripped abs and big biceps?

All things work.

That's it.

All things work to some degree in some fashion for some period of time.

You see, the body is a wonderfully adaptive machine. It is the product of millions of years of evolution. Your body was meant to survive very harsh conditions, everything from famine to war. If you push your body to its limits, then it has no choice but to adapt. It's only other choice would be to die.

So if you push your body to its extreme and do it consistently and safely, then it has no choice but to lose fat and grow stronger and bigger, even in the midst of physical stress.

Personal trainers know this, whether consciously or unconsciously. If you can do 50 pushups, then a personal trainer will simply order you to do 100 pushups. Most personal trainers don't have any special wisdom or scientific knowledge. They simply push you harder and harder and push your pain threshold higher and higher.

The trainees who are willing to take punishment day in and day out are the ones who end up on infomercials with the before and after pictures. The ones who quit? They're selling their P90X DVD's on Craig's List.

The secret to success is not the program. The secret to success is your commitment to the program. For every successful physique transformation there are thousands who quit after the first workout. Infomercials highlight the success stories, not the failures.

Just because all things work, however, doesn't mean all things work forever. People always want the perfect program, one that will give results all the time. But if you stick with an exercise program long enough, then you will eventually hit a wall. You'll stop losing fat, and you'll stop gaining muscle.

Remember: your body is a highly adaptive machine. Given enough time it will adapt to any exercise program and any diet. And because the human body is adaptive, there is no "perfect program." The perfect exercise program is change. The perfect program is a variety of programs.

This is why it's important to know that an exercise program not only works, but why it works and how it works. If you know how and why something works, then you'll know when to use it and for what purpose.

There are three things you will learn in this book:

1) Bodybuilding is a process of building then refining, isolating then integrating. You will learn what exercises build muscle over your entire musculature and what exercises target specific muscle groups.
2) High muscular tension is THE primary growth factor. All other training parameters (weight, reps, sets, tempo, exercises, etc.) are manipulations of this factor in training. You will learn what exercises produce high muscular tension, and you will learn how to manipulate the intensity and the duration of tension to achieve muscle size and tone.
3) Microcycling and backcycling are the keys to sustained muscular growth and size. Your body is highly adaptive, so developing a complete physique means you need variety: a variety of exercises, a variety of training programs. This variety needs to be cycled, however, in order to sustain muscular size and achieve muscular growth.

This latest volume of Strength and Physique will provide you with a variety of exercises and a variety of exercise strategies.   This book will dissect and analyze the mechanisms of muscle growth, so that you'll understand how and why an exercise program is effective.

This book will give you the knowledge and programs to transform your body. All you need to bring to the table is unwavering commitment.

Build then Refine

I. Build Then Refine

What's your goal as a bodybuilder? Are you looking to simply get bigger? Or are you looking to put on muscle in specific body parts? Is your goal "symmetry" or is it "bulk?"

To develop muscle bulk a trainee builds as much muscle as possible throughout his body, regardless of how it looks overall. This concept is also known as "power bodybuilding," whereby you develop muscle mass through the use of heavy compound (multi-joint) movements (bench press, rows, military press, deadlifts and squats) with some supplementary bodybuilding movements (barbell curls, lateral raises, lying triceps extensions).

There is a problem with the power bodybuilding method: if you want to look good naked and appeal to the opposite sex, then this method alone will not give you that look. The heavy compound movements build mass over your musculature, but they build muscle indiscriminately. Power bodybuilding is analogous to using a shotgun to destroy your target. It's not pretty, but it gets the job done.

Heavy compound movements such as bench presses, back squats and deadlifts develop a thick and stocky look. Deadlifts build up the trapezius, which detracts from the wide shoulder look sought after by bodybuilders. Heavy benching build up the chest, but you'll end up with man boobs.

Despite their well-developed six packs, a lot of power bodybuilders have distended guts. This is due to a combination of overeating and heavy squatting. In order to squat heavy, a power bodybuilder needs to fill his diaphragm with air and expand his waistline in order to create a stable base from which to lift. Heavy squats as well as heavy deadlifts will thicken the hips and build up the glutes, which takes away from the long legged look desired by many bodybuilders, particularly those of smaller stature.

This is not to say power bodybuilding moves should be avoided completely. Movements such as deadlifts and squats can be used to add much needed mass on an ectomorph, and the mass can be refined through the use of more targeted bodybuilding movements. If you're an endomorph or a mesomorph, however, then you should forego bulking up to gain muscle. Focus on developing "muscle symmetry" instead.

Muscle Symmetry

Muscle symmetry is the idea that a bodybuilder develops muscle in *certain* body parts to create a physique that is pleasing to the eye. This physique aesthetic is known as a "V-taper" or an "X-frame," and it is characterized by broad shoulders and a narrow waist, and long toned legs. The V-taper or X-frame is the hallmark of the "classical bodybuilder."

For the classical bodybuilder, particular exercises are performed to target and develop particular muscles and particular portions of a muscle complex. Rather than use the "shotgun approach" of power bodybuilders, classical bodybuilders use a targeted approach to muscle building. Strategic muscles are developed to give the overall illusion of size, while the development of other body parts is minimized to obtain the ideal shoulder to waist ratio. Classical bodybuilders focus on these areas of the body:

- Broad shoulders, with minimal trapezius development
- V-tapered back, with special emphasis on the teres major
- Thick, wide tapered chest shaped like this _|_/ not this (_|_)
- Small, flat waist
- Narrow hips and minimal glute development
- Long toned legs, with special emphasis on the vastus medialis and calves
- Thick muscular arms

To forge the ideal physique, a classical bodybuilder will focus on developing his "pivot point" muscles. The term pivot points was coined by Lou Degni and brought to public attention by Larry Scott. The concept is that certain muscles are located in strategic points of the body and that development of these muscles will create an august muscular physique which stresses muscularity and V-taper:

1. Calves
2. Lateral deltoid
3. Triceps long head
4. Brachialis (under the biceps)
5. Posterior deltoid
6. Upper chest
7. Vastus medialis (quadriceps)
8. Teres major (back)
9. Forearms

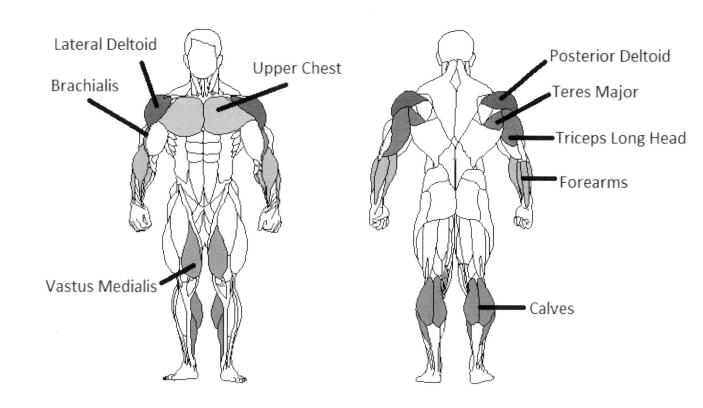

The 9 Pivot Point Muscles

As you can see, pivot points are typically located at the extremities (such as the calves and forearms) and near joints. Development of these areas emphasizes the overall look of muscularity, even if the lifter's physique is lightweight and trim. A classic example of the pivot point physique is Frank Zane.

Think of pivot point training as investing: if you only had so much money to invest, then you want to invest it in stocks, businesses, or properties with the greatest returns. Likewise, if your goal were simply to look good for the beach or for a movie role, then you would concentrate your training on muscles that give your physique the most visual bang for your buck. For bodybuilders whose goals are cosmetic, pivot point training is a solid strategy to follow and provides a clearly defined set of training goals.

Development of each pivot point, however, requires an understanding of each body part's training personality: What exercises target the pivot point? What set extension techniques best develop the pivot point? Is the pivot point fast-twitch or slow-twitch dominant? In later chapters of this book, we'll discuss each muscle group's pivot point and how to fully develop it.

Establish Your Goal: Symmetry or Bulk?

Bodybuilding is always a process of building muscle and then refining that muscle. You build muscular bulk through power bodybuilding exercises and then you refine your muscle through classical bodybuilding exercises. It's like sculpting: you can't shape or mold what you don't have. You have to add on the "clay" or muscle and then take away some of that clay to shape and refine the muscle.

If you're an endomorph or a mesomorph, then focus on classical bodybuilding movements. Focus on getting ripped through strength training and sculpting and refining the muscle you already have. Focus on developing your pivot points for ultimate muscularity.

If you're an ectomorph, then you have a longer road ahead of you. You have to build muscle first. You may be tempted to train like others and include 4-5 different exercises for each body part. For an ectomorph, however, you have to build muscle by first building up your strength. To be strong you have to focus on mastering a few select exercises.

The following are power bodybuilding exercises to build size and strength over your entire musculature. The first 3 exercises (clean and press, deadlifts, squats) are what I call "anabolic blowtorches." These exercises provoke a huge dump of testosterone in your system and stimulate total body hypertrophy:

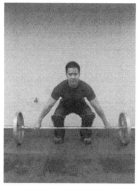 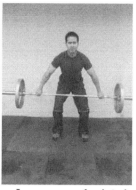 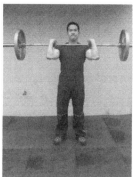 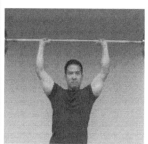

Barbell clean and press (which can be broken down into 2 movements: hang cleans and standing military presses)

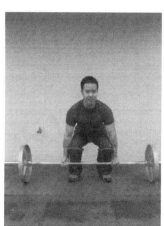 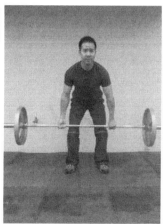 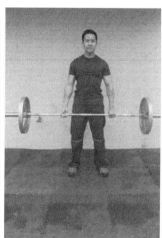

Deadlifts

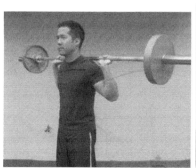 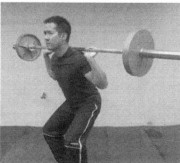 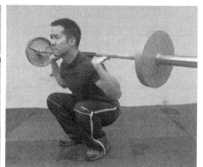

Back squats

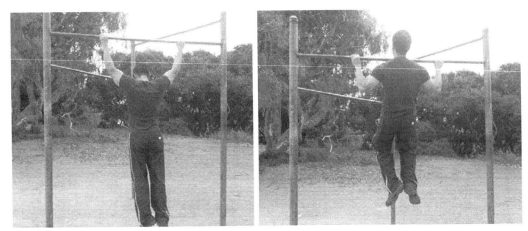

Pull-ups

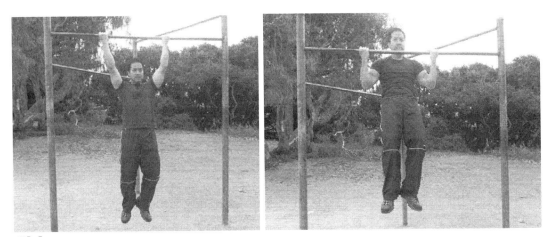

Chin-ups

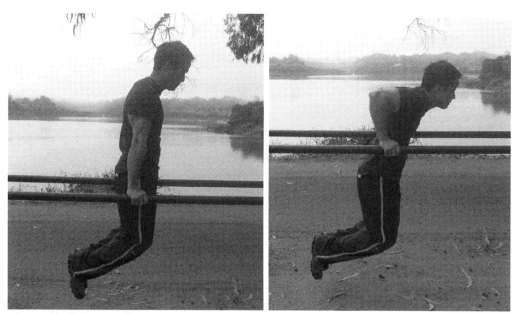

Parallel bar dips

The Power Bodybuilding Program

If you are an ectomorph and are in need of muscle bulk, then the following program will help you build it. The program incorporates the anabolic blowtorches and is meant to help ectomorphs put on weight and develop strength. Advanced bodybuilders, however, can use this program to "back cycle" or scale back on their training.

Monday	Wednesday	Friday
Clean and Press: • 3 sets, 3-6 reps • 3 minutes rest **Pull-ups:** • 2 sets, as many reps as possible • 3 minutes rest **Deadlifts:** • 3 sets, 3-6 reps • 3 minutes **Parallel Bar Dips:** • 2 sets, as many reps as possible • 3 minutes rest	**Hang Cleans:** • 3 sets, 3-6 reps • 3 minutes rest **Chin-ups:** • 2 sets, as many reps as possible • 3 minutes rest **Parallel Bar Dips:** • 2 sets, as many reps as possible • 3 minutes rest **Military Press:** • 3 sets, 10-12 reps • 3 minutes rest	**Clean and Press:** • 3 sets, 3-6 reps • 3 minutes rest **Pull-ups:** • 2 sets, as many reps as possible • 3 minutes rest **Squats:** • 3 sets, 10-12 reps • 3 minutes rest **Parallel Bar Dips:** • 2 sets, as many reps as possible • 3 minutes rest

When performing the exercises, choose weights that allow you to comfortably perform the recommended reps. In other words, do not go to absolute muscular failure. For example, choose a 7-8 rep max weight to perform the recommended 3-6 reps in good form. Up the weight only if you can perform the recommended reps with relative ease. Be conservative at first when estimating what weight to use.

If you cannot perform pull-ups, chin-ups or dips, then you may substitute pulldowns and bench presses. Perform 3 sets of 10-12 reps for bench presses and pulldowns.

HOWEVER, if you can perform at least 3 full range pull-ups or 3 full range dips, then you must perform pull-ups, chin-ups or dips. You need to develop an underlying base of strength in order to gain more muscle, and difficult bodyweight exercises develop real world strength far better than machines. DO NOT PERFORM PULL-UPS OR DIPS ON A MACHINE.

Follow the program for 3-6 weeks. Then switch to a different program of your choosing, preferably a program with higher reps. Come back to the program whenever you need to bulk up. Be sure to eat a lot of food during this bulking program.

Key Points on Symmetry and Bulk:

- If you're an ectomorph, then you must build muscular bulk through power bodybuilding exercises.
- If you're a mesomorph or endomorph, then you must refine your muscle through bodybuilding exercises that target your pivot points. Focus on developing symmetry.

High Tension Exercises:
The Key to Muscular Growth

II. High Tension Exercises: The Key to Muscle Growth

In this book are exercise combinations and training principles that I've used on myself and my clients to develop the classical bodybuilder look. Some of the exercises will be familiar to you and are standard exercises used in most bodybuilding regimens. Other exercises will be rather esoteric and unconventional. These exercises are rarely seen in the gym, because they are difficult to learn and require greater coordination. They were largely forgotten once machines took over more and more space in the gym.

The exercises showcased are primarily free weights: barbells, dumbbells, kettlebells and bodyweight exercises. Although machines can grow muscle, they just do not grow as much muscle as free weight exercises. Free weights beat machines for developing size and strength, period. Machines stabilize the weight for you, so you end up using less muscle to push or pull the weight. Free weights, however, force you to perfect your form and to stabilize your body while pushing or pulling the weight. This greater engagement of your muscles means greater activation and greater growth.

Most people choose machines, because they choose the easy way out in everything. But if you want an uncommon physique, then don't take the easy way out. Quit the machines and do free weights: barbells, dumbbells, kettlebells and bodyweight.

Free weight exercises also add a lot of variety to your training regimen. With a machine you're stuck performing an exercise in only one position. With free weights, however, the same exercise can be done in multiple ways:

- By varying the angle of your body or bench
- By varying the type of grip: overhand, underhand or neutral grip
- By varying the width of your grip: wide, shoulder-width, narrow

A single exercise can be done in multiple ways with free weights. An overhead press can be done as a barbell military press, a dumbbell Scott press, a kettlebell clean and press or as a handstand pushup.

I have included the exercises in this book, because these exercises grow muscle. The exercises will either produce mass over your entire musculature or they will grow a targeted muscle group. The reason these exercises work can be summed up in one word: tension.

High Tension is the Key to Muscular Growth

Studies and anecdotal evidence show that wrestlers, Olympic weightlifters, powerlifters, gymnasts and bodybuilders all develop significant amounts muscle through seemingly different training modalities. The common factor in the training modalities of all of these athletes (if you call bodybuilders athletes) is HIGH MUSCULAR TENSION.

Each of these athletes produces high muscular tension in their training through different means. Wrestlers create tension in their muscles by wrestling with each other. Gymnasts create high muscular tension by performing extremely difficult bodyweight exercises on the pommel horse, hanging rings and parallel bars.

Olympic weightlifters, powerlifters and bodybuilders use barbells in their training, but each group differs in their use of barbells. Weightlifters lift explosively. Their exercises (the clean and jerk, the snatch) produce high but brief amounts of tension. Powerlifters focus on slow strength, and hence their exercises (bench press, deadlift and squat) produce high amounts of tension for a longer duration.

Bodybuilders lift moderately heavy weights in comparison to powerlifters and weightlifters, but they focus on higher reps and extended sets on a wide variety of exercises. The duration of muscular tension that bodybuilders produce when they lift is much longer, and this is part of the reason why bodybuilders, as a whole, have larger, leaner muscles than powerlifters or Olympic lifters.

Muscular tension is the key to growth. The more tension you can create within a muscle, the more size you will incur. The tension has to be high (heavy weight), and it has to be of the right duration (at least 20 seconds or at least 5 reps). Furthermore the tension on the muscle should be consistently strong throughout the entire range of motion of the exercise.

Let's take the triceps kickback for example. The tension is low throughout much of the range of motion, with the exception of the very top where you flex the triceps. Yet this upper range of tension is so brief (1-2 seconds), it doesn't do much for muscular hypertrophy. Not only that, but you can't use much weight in the triceps kickback, which cuts down the tension even further. So there's a lack of muscular tension by weight, duration and range of motion.

Now if we choose exercises that create high muscular tension, for a long duration and throughout the entire range of motion, then you can easily incur size on just a few sets per muscle group.

Very few exercises (namely pull-ups) maintain high tension on a muscle throughout its entire range. Muscular tension varies along the range of motion for the vast majority of exercises. To compensate for these gaps in tension, it's best to hit a muscle group from multiple angles.

The exercises found in this book will produce high tension in a targeted muscle group or within your entire musculature. Some will produce more tension for a longer duration than others. Few exercises will produce high muscular throughout the entire range of motion, while most exercises will produce high tension at only specific points of their ranges of motion. Exercises which produce this partial range of tension can be paired or grouped with other exercises to approximate a full range of muscular tension. The chapters on body part training will teach you how to aggregate exercises in such a manner.

I have not included every exercise variation in this book. I have included only those exercises which produce high muscular tension. These exercises will either build mass over your entire musculature or they will target specific pivot points that enhance the classical bodybuilder look. Variations can be made of each of these exercises by varying your grip and angle of execution.

All exercises work muscle, but not all exercises *build* muscle. The exercises in this book are meant to build muscle and to build muscle in all the right places.

Key Points on Muscular Tension:

- Free weight exercises are better than machines for muscular growth.
- High muscular tension is the key to muscular growth.
- Muscular tension must be:
  - High (use heavy weight)
  - Long (the set should be at least 20 seconds in duration or at least 5 reps)
  - Throughout the entire range of motion

Fiber Type and Reps

III. Fiber Type and Reps

If high muscular tension stimulates muscle growth, then how do you determine the amount of tension needed to induce hypertrophy? What weight do you choose? How do you determine the minimal time under tension that the muscle must endure in order to grow? How many reps should you perform?

To determine the intensity and duration of the muscular tension needed to grow, you must determine the fiber make-up of the muscle being worked. Some muscles are composed primarily of fast-twitch fibers; some are composed of slow-twitch fibers.

Whether a muscle is predominantly fast-twitch or slow-twitch determines the range of repetitions the muscle should perform in order to grow. Fiber type also determines the "tempo" or speed in which you should be performing a rep.

Fast-twitch muscles are designed for speed, strength and power (a combination of speed and strength). Fast-twitch muscle fibers have a high potential for growth. Fast-twitch muscles respond best to lower reps (1-9) and heavy weight. Fast-twitch muscles grow through the explosive lifting (concentric) and the controlled lowering (eccentric) of the weight being lifted.

Slow-twitch muscles are designed for endurance and have a lower potential for growth. They respond best to light weight and high reps (10+). With slow-twitch muscles, the number of reps is more important than the amount of weight used. In order to perform a high number of reps, you have to use a brisk tempo. Hence, slow-twitch muscles respond best to a quick concentric with almost no eccentric emphasis.

Mixed fiber muscles respond to a wide variety of tempos and reps, because these muscle groups have an equal amount of fast and slow-twitch muscle fiber. Mixed fiber muscles can lift fast or slow, high reps or low reps, and they will grow either way.

By understanding the fiber make-up of each muscle group, you can determine the number of reps that each muscle should be performing in order to grow. By determining the ideal number of repetitions, you determine both the intensity of the tension (the weight lifted) and the duration of the tension (the number of repetitions).

For example, if you know that the long head of the triceps consists of predominantly fast-twitch muscle fibers, then you know it grows best on heavy weight and low reps. If the triceps long head responds best to a rep range of 4-6, then you know how much weight to use (your 6 rep maximum) and you know how many reps to perform (4-6) to develop the fast-twitch fibers. You also know that with each repetition you must lift the weight explosively and slowly lower the weight under control.

Very few people are purely fast-twitch or purely slow-twitch. Although there can be wide variations among people regarding their muscle fiber make-up, in general most people have the following muscle group compositions:

Muscle Group	Fiber Makeup	Rep range
Chest	Mixed	Continuum: 3-20+ reps Target: 6-10 reps
Back	Latissimus dorsi: Mixed	Continuum: 3-20+ reps Target: 6-10 reps
	Teres major: Slow-twitch	Continuum: 8-20+ reps Target: 10-15 reps
Deltoids	Anterior: Fast-twitch	Continuum: 3-10+ reps Target: 4-6 reps
	Lateral: Slow-twitch	Continuum: 8-20+ reps Target: 10-15 reps
	Posterior: Mixed	Continuum: 6-20+ reps Target: 6-10 reps
Quadriceps	Mixed	Continuum: 3-20+ reps Target: 6-10 reps
Hamstrings	Biceps femoris: fast-twitch	Continuum: 3-8 reps Target: 4-6 reps
	Semitendinosus, semimembranosus: mixed fiber makeup	Continuum: 3-12+ reps Target: 4-6 reps
Biceps	Biceps brachii: mixed fiber makeup	Continuum: 3-15+ reps Target: 6-10 reps
	Brachialis: fast-twitch	Continuum: 3-8 reps Target: 4-6 reps
Triceps	Long Head: fast-twitch	Continuum: 3-8 reps Target: 4-6 reps
	Lateral and Medial heads: mixed fiber makeup	Continuum: 3-20+ reps Target: 4-6 reps
Calves	Gastrocnemius: fast-twitch	Continuum: 6-20+ reps Target: 6-10 reps
	Soleus: slow-twitch	Continuum: 10-40+ reps Target: 10-25 reps
Abdominals	Fast-twitch	Continuum: 3-20+ reps Target: 4-10 reps
Forearms	Slow-twitch	Continuum: 4-25+ reps Target: 10-25 reps

Note: The plus sign (+) means "and beyond." 20+ translates to "20 reps and beyond."

Each muscle group has a continuum of reps, a range of repetitions that you can perform to achieve hypertrophy. How broad the rep continuum is will depend on the muscle. If you're interested in full muscular hypertrophy, then you must perform a wide variety of reps within the muscle's rep continuum.

Within the rep continuum is a target rep range, one that the muscle responds to best due to its fiber makeup. While it's important to know the target rep range for a muscle group, you shouldn't train exclusively in that rep bracket, since there are other fibers with potential for growth. To fully develop a muscle, you should cycle your reps within the muscle's rep continuum. The bulk of your training, however, will be in the target rep range.

Muscles that are primarily fast-twitch (such as the hamstrings and the long head of the triceps) tend to have very narrow rep continuums. Slow-twitch muscles (such as the soleus muscle of the calf) and mixed fiber muscles (such as the chest, biceps, quads, and back) will have broad rep continuums. So while your hamstrings have a narrow rep continuum (3-8), your quadriceps muscles have a broad rep continuum (3-20).

Since mixed fiber muscles respond to very broad rep continuums, they will grow on varying tempos and a wide variety of reps. Muscles that are pure fast-twitch or pure slow-twitch, however, require very specific training parameters. The three muscles that stand out in this regard are the deltoid lateral head (slow-twitch), triceps (fast-twitch) and hamstrings (fast-twitch). These three muscles each have very distinct "personalities" and will only grow in response to their specific rep ranges and tempos.

In later chapters, we'll discuss each muscle group and its unique personality. We'll discuss high tension exercises for each muscle group. We'll also examine each muscle group's fiber make-up and the ideal tempo and rep ranges for growth.

Exploit Fast-Twitch Fibers for Maximum Growth

If you are new to weight training or if you are performing an exercise for the first time, then you should start with light weights and execute higher reps (10+) regardless of the fiber makeup of the muscles being worked. Your muscles and in particular your nervous system need to repeatedly practice an exercise in order to become stronger at it. In order to practice the exercise, you have to repeatedly execute the exercise through high repetition. This is why beginners respond best to the 8-12 rep range.

Once you have been training consistently for some time, however, your muscles will no longer respond to 10+ reps or even 8+ reps. Your muscles and your nervous system will get stronger and stronger and will crave heavier and heavier weights in order to grow. Over the years, your training will naturally shift from high repetitions (8-12) to low repetitions (3-8) from heavy weight.

The heavier the weight: the greater the tension on the muscles being worked. The greater the muscular tension, the greater the muscular hypertrophy. Remember, it is tension that causes the targeted muscle fibers to thicken up and get bigger. Heavy weight and low reps exploit the fast-twitch muscle fibers, which grow much larger than their high rep, slow-twitch counterparts.

This shift from high reps to low reps is a natural evolution in your training. Your body wants the biggest bang for its buck. It wants to maximize its training efforts, and the greatest hypertrophic response will come from fast-twitch muscle fibers. More fast-twitch fiber means far more muscular growth and size.

You can train your muscles to be more fast-twitch. Mixed fiber muscle groups (chest, back, biceps, quads) will shift their compositions to fast-twitch fibers the longer you train them with low reps and heavy weight. Even slow-twitch muscles (calves, forearms and deltoids) will grow on lower repetitions, since slow-twitch dominant muscles still have some fast-twitch fibers. The soleus calf muscle is 80% slow-twitch, so there is a significant 20% of the soleus that is fast-twitch. That's 20% of potential growth!

Active Recovery Sets

If you stick solely to low reps, however, then you will stagnate on them as well. Although the tension is high with heavy weight and low reps, the tension is not very long in duration with repetitions below 6. Training heavily with low reps is a solid way to gain size, but eventually those size gains will come to a screeching halt if you train on low reps exclusively.

Heavy weight and low reps will hypertrophy the fast-twitch muscle fibers. Over time, however, these fibers will thicken up and crowd each other. Very little blood will flow into these fibers, and nutrients and hormones will not reach them easily.

To continue grow, you have to pump and flush the muscles with blood. You have to switch back to higher reps. The high rep pump promotes growth by developing the capillaries and circulating blood into the muscles being worked. This blood circulation will transport anabolic hormones and nutrients into the muscles, as well as transport out toxins left over from your previous workouts.

Periodically performing higher reps to facilitate recovery and growth is known as "active recovery." People from different bodybuilding and powerlifting camps have called high rep active recovery sets by various names, such as feeder sets, flushing sets, pump sets, etc.

Active recovery sets are light sets of 12 reps and beyond (15, 20, etc.) that pump blood into your muscles to flush out the lingering waste by-products (indicated by muscle soreness) from the last workout and to transport in nutrients and circulating hormones to facilitate recovery and growth. If you are sore from your last workout, then you can literally work the soreness out with a few high rep active recovery sets.

Thus it is important to "periodize" or cycle between high reps and low reps throughout the week. If you want to get big and strong, then develop the fast-twitch muscle fibers by focusing on lower reps (3-8), but throw in some active recovery sets every third workout. This is why it is important to understand a muscle's rep continuum, since you'll know the upper limit of reps in which you can train a muscle for active recovery.

If you train each body part 3 times per week, then the ratio of low rep/fast-twitch workouts to high rep/active recovery workouts should be 2:1. Two workouts should consist of lower reps (3-8); one workout should consist of higher reps (8+) with some active recovery sets (12+ reps). A set and rep pattern of 3-4 sets of 12-15+ reps, 30-60 seconds rest periods, done once a week should be fine.

Active recovery sets are the key to high frequency training. Active recovery sets speed up recovery, and they facilitate growth. They allow you to train more frequently, and training more frequently allows you gain muscle at a faster rate.

Key Points on Reps:

- Fiber type determines the number of repetitions and the tempo of lifting required for muscle growth.
- If you are new to weight training or if you are performing an exercise for the first time, then you should start with light weights and execute higher reps (8-12) regardless of the muscle's fiber composition.
- Over the years, your training will naturally shift from high repetitions (8-12) to low repetitions (3-8) from heavy weight. Your muscles will become fast-twitch dominant.
- Cycle your reps within the muscle's rep continuum by doing some active recovery workouts. The ratio of low rep/fast-twitch workouts to high rep/active recovery workouts should be 2:1.

Manipulating Tempo to Increase Muscular Tension

IV. Manipulating Tempo to Increase Muscular Tension

What is tempo? Tempo is the speed of a repetition. Tempo refers to how quickly you lift and lower the weight. Lifting the weight is called the concentric or positive portion of the rep. Lowering the weight is called the eccentric or negative portion of the rep.

Different tempos will have different effects on muscle. Explosive reps activate the fast-twitch fibers and increase insulin sensitivity in the muscles being worked. Slow negative reps will release localized hormones Insulin Growth Factor (IGF) and Fibroblast Growth Factor (FGF), both potent anabolic hormones. Flexing a muscle in its fully contracted position will increase myogenic tone. Stretching a muscle at the bottom of the rep will increase androgen receptors in the muscle itself. ?

So what is the ideal tempo for gaining muscular size?

As a general catch all rule, the ideal tempo is a fast explosive rep, since this tempo preferentially develops the big fast-twitch muscle fibers. Explosive lifting generates a higher level of force production within the muscles being worked. High force production from the muscle equals to greater tension on the muscle.

Whether or not you use slow negatives depends on the exercise. Although slow negatives increase both the intensity and duration of muscular tension, some exercises simply don't allow for slow negatives without a reduction in weight. Certain kettlebell exercises and Olympic lifts can only be done explosively with no negative emphasis.

Tempo is always tricky, because tempo depends on the mechanics of the exercise and the muscle group being worked.

Say you're doing dumbbell rows. The ideal tempo would be "explosive lift, quick drop." In other words, fast positive, fast negative, no pauses. The mechanics of the exercise don't allow you to do slow negatives and prolonged contractions without dropping the amount of weight, which would drop the amount of force generated and reduce the tension on the muscle.

On the other hand, if you're doing lying leg curls, then your tempo might look like this: fast positive, contract hard for 2 seconds, slow negative and no pause at bottom. The mechanics of the leg curl machine exercise allow you to perform explosive reps with accentuated negative reps.

Bottom line is that tempo will depend on what exercise you're performing. It's the interaction of the mechanics of the exercise and the fiber make-up of the muscles worked that determines the ideal tempo for size and strength.

Fiber Type	Reps	Tempo
Fast-twitch muscles	1-6 reps	Explosive Lifts (i.e. Olympic lifts, kettlebells): fast positive, fast negative Slow Lifts (i.e. powerlifting, bodybuilding): fast positive, slow negative
Mixed fiber muscles	All reps but shoot for a target range of 6-10 reps	fast positive, fast or slow negative
Slow-twitch muscles	10+ reps	fast positive, fast negative

Keep in mind that the heavier the weight, the slower you may be performing the reps. This is the case with near maximal weights. You may try to lift your 3 rep maximum explosively, but the weight is moving slowly because it is so heavy.

What is important is not the actual speed of the lift, but that your muscles are generating maximum explosive force underneath the bar. The actual speed of the lift is going to be slow with heavy loads, but it's the intent to move the weight explosively that matters.

Also keep in mind that if a slow negative tempo is required, you will slow down that portion of the rep and resist the pull of the weight. A good rule of thumb for slow negatives is to extend the lowering of the weight to 3-5 seconds.

Regardless of the speed, always lift in good form. Perform the exercises correctly and safely. If your form starts to break down or the speed of your lift starts to slow down, then it is time to end the set. There is no point in performing extra reps, if those reps are of poor quality. You are more likely to get injured from doing extra reps with sloppy form.

Some of the exercise descriptions in this book will recommend a tempo recommendation designed to maximize tension on the muscles being worked.

Key Points on Tempo:

- Tempo is always tricky, because tempo depends on the mechanics of the exercise and the muscle group being worked.
- The ideal tempo is a fast explosive rep, since this tempo preferentially develops the big fast-twitch muscle fibers.
- The actual speed of the lift is going to be slow with heavy loads, but it's the intent to move the weight explosively that matters.

Extending Muscular Tension

V. Extending Muscular Tension

As mentioned in previous chapters, fast-twitch muscles fibers have a higher potential for growth than their slow-twitch counterparts. You will get a bigger bang for your buck if your training is focused on developing the fast-twitch fibers.

The reason fast-twitch muscle fibers have a high potential for growth is that they respond best to heavy weight. So when you choose a weight with which you can only perform 6 reps, then you know that the muscular tension generated from lifting your 6 rep max (6RM) is very high compared to lifting your 12 rep max (12RM).

The problem is that although the muscular tension is high, the time under tension is brief at 6 reps. To fully grow you want to stress your muscles with high tension for a longer duration of time. You want the high muscular tension generated from a 6RM, but you want to maintain that high tension for the duration of a 12RM.

You can overcome short durations of tension by *extending the set.* Set extension techniques are techniques whereby you perform a set close to muscular failure and then perform another set immediately afterward to work the same muscle group.

With set extenders you can maintain high muscular tension for a longer duration. Maintaining high muscular tension for a long duration grows a lot of muscle and grows muscle fairly quickly.

The following are set extenders you can use in the gym:

Cluster Reps. This is a variation of the rest-pause method. With the traditional rest-pause method, you take 90% of your 1RM, perform 1 rep, rest 10-15 seconds, perform 1 rep, rest 10-15 seconds, so on and so forth until you've completed 6-8 reps.

With cluster reps, the number reps are higher and more varied. Since the volume (number of reps) is higher with cluster reps, this technique is much more conducive to muscle growth than regular rest-pause.

To perform cluster reps, take a weight where you can only perform half of the required reps. In rest-pause fashion, you will perform as many reps as you can, stop and rest briefly, resume the set and crank out more reps, stop and rest briefly. You keep repeating this process until you've achieved the desired number of reps.

For example, if the program calls for 16 cluster reps of close grip bench presses, then your performance may look like this:

- Load up your 8RM
- You perform 7 reps, stopping just short of failure
- You rack the weight and rest for 10-15 seconds
- You resume the set and crank out 4 more reps
- You rest for 10-15 seconds
- You resume the set and perform 3 more reps
- You rest for 10-15 seconds
- You crank out the last 2 reps and reach your target of 16 reps

Essentially you are performing mini-sets with mini-rests in between. Keep cranking out reps and resting until you reach the target number. Cluster reps are an excellent way of increasing time under tension without reducing the weight. This makes it an ideal set extension technique for mixed fiber and fast-twitch dominant muscles.

Diminishing Sets. A high rep variation of cluster reps is known as "diminishing sets." With diminishing sets, you choose a weight and strive to perform a total of 100 reps in the fewest number of sets possible.

Typically, bodyweight exercises such as dips, pushups and pull-ups are chosen when performing diminishing sets. Since you're performing a high number of reps with each set, diminishing sets hypertrophy the slow-twitch endurance fibers.

So if you were performing diminishing sets of pushups, then your reps may look like this:

Set 1- 30 reps
Set 2- 20 reps
Set 3- 15 reps
Set 4- 15 reps
Set 5- 10 reps
Set 6- 10 reps

The next time you perform diminishing sets you will strive to hit 100 reps in fewer than 6 sets.

Descending sets. While cluster reps work best for fast-twitch and mixed fiber muscles, descending sets work best for mixed fiber and slow-twitch muscles, such as the lateral (medial) deltoid and calves. This technique also works best in a commercial gym, where you can easily implement it on a dumbbell rack or a cable machine. Simply choose a weight, perform a set, then drop down to the next weight and immediately perform another set. Keep dropping weight and performing sets until you reach your desired total number of sets and reps.

So if you were to perform descending sets of lateral raises, then your poundage and reps may look similar to this:

Set 1- 25 pounds, 10 reps, no rest
Set 2- 20 pounds, 8 reps, no rest
Set 3- 15 pounds, 6 reps, no rest
Set 4- 10 pounds, 6 reps

Compound sets. This is when you perform two exercises in a row for one body part. Compound sets are different from supersets, where you alternate between sets of two different body parts. Compound sets can be implemented in three ways:

- The Post-Exhaust Compound Set- If you're a bodybuilding enthusiast, then you've heard of the pre-exhaust method. Well, the post-exhaust compound set is the exact opposite. Post-exhaust requires that you perform a multi-joint movement for a body part followed by a single-joint movement for that same body part. An example of this would be a pull-up followed by stiff-arm pulldowns.

- The Heavy/Light Compound Set- This is where you perform low reps with heavy weight for one exercise, then immediately perform higher reps with a lighter weight of another exercise. The heavy/light method can be combined with the post-exhaust method: front squats (4-6 reps) followed immediately by leg extensions (10-12 reps).

- Bifurcated Compound Set- This is when you pair 2 exercises to stress both sides of a muscle group. Most exercises tend to stress one portion of the muscle group over the other. Very few exercises will stress the entire muscle group evenly. In terms of achieving full muscular development, the bifurcated compound set is the most important version of the compound set.

Muscle Group		
Chest	Upper Chest • Neck press • 20º bench press • Feet elevated pushups	Lower Chest • Dips
Back	Latissimus Dorsi, Teres Major (Back Width) • Pull-ups • Chin-ups • Pulldowns	Midback (Back Thickness) • Dumbbell rows • Cable rows • Deadlifts • Power cleans
Deltoids	Lateral Deltoid • Lateral raises • Swing laterals • Lean away laterals • Wide grip upright rows • Barbell high pulls	Posterior Deltoid • Side lying rear flyes Anterior Deltoid* • Military press • Clean and Press • Scott press *The anterior deltoid is recruited in all pressing movements, including those for the chest. For this reason, anterior deltoid exercises are not included in compound sets.
Biceps	Biceps Brachii • Lying dumbbell curls • Incline curls • Concentration curls • Body drag curls • Perfect curls	Brachialis (Biceps Peak) • Zottman curls • Incline hammer curls • Preacher curls • Reverse grip curls
Triceps	Triceps Long Head • Lying EZ-curl bar extensions • Decline EZ-curl bar extensions	Triceps Lateral Head, Triceps Medial Head • Lying dumbbell extensions • Decline dumbbell extensions • Dips • Pushups

		• Overhead press
Quadriceps	Vastus Medialis ("Tear drop") • Front squats • Hack squats • Sissy squats	Vastus Lateralis, Rectus Femoris • Reverse lunges • One-legged squats
Hamstrings	Biceps Femoris • Standing one-legged curl • Seated leg curls • Lying leg curls	Semitendinosus, Semimembranosus • Romanian deadlifts • Good mornings
Calves	Gastrocnemius • Dumbbell calf raise • One legged calf raise	Soleus • Seated calf raise
Abdominals	Rectus Abdominus (Six-Pack) • Hanging leg raises • Dragon flags	Transverse Abdominus • Stomach vacuums • Planks

Trisets. This is when you string together 3 exercises for the same muscle group. Suppose you can do pull-ups, but you can only perform 4-6 reps. You can extend the set for your back by doing a triset such as this:

- Pull-ups (4-6 reps)
- Dumbbell pullovers (6-8 reps)
- Stiff-arm lat pulldowns (6-8 reps)

Instead of just doing a set of 4-6 reps, you've now done a triset of 14-20 reps for the back. This is another great way to increase time under tension on a muscle.

The other advantage of this technique is that you can string together 3 different exercises to stress the entire *force curve*.

"Use the Force Curve, Luke!"

A force curve (also known as a strength curve) is a graphical representation of the muscular force generated at each point throughout an exercise's range of motion. Because of joint angles, the resistance or tension of an exercise is not constant. The tension varies throughout the exercise movement.

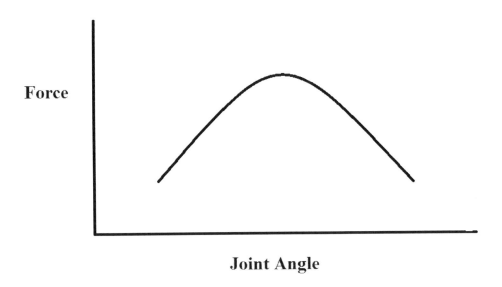

Let's use the biceps curl as an example. When you curl, you will feel the weight or the tension more or less at various points of the biceps curl. The force curve will be different for different biceps curl variations.

If you do preacher curls, then the bottom range of the movement will be the hardest portion to work through, because the resistance is greatest there. If you do barbell curls, then the tension is greatest midrange. And if you do spider curls, then the tension is greatest at the top range in the fully contracted position.

To fully maximize tension on a muscle throughout its entire range of motion, you can construct a triset of three exercises, each stressing a different strength curve: top range, midrange, bottom range.

Biceps Triset:

1. Spider Curls (top range)
2. Standing Barbell Curls (middle range)
3. Preacher Curls (bottom range)

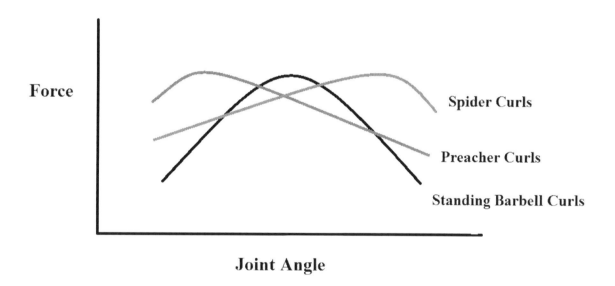

By aggregating 3 different exercises with complementary strength curves, you can create high muscular tension throughout the entire range of motion. You'll get an incredible pump when you perform trisets in such a manner. This is not simply because you're performing a lot of reps. Maximizing tension throughout a muscle's entire range of motion activates a greater number of muscle fibers than stressing only one force curve.

In the later chapters of this book, I will show you the strength curves of different exercises and show you how to combine various exercises to maximize muscular tension throughout the entire range of motion.

How to Perform Set Extenders in a Commercial Gym

While you can perform descending sets and cluster reps with a single piece of gym equipment, trisets and compound sets require greater setup. Anyone who has tried to perform a triset or a superset in a commercial gym knows how pissed off people can be when you hog up multiple pieces of equipment. Plus people will jump in on a machine, thinking that you're done because you moved on to the next exercise.

If you want to perform set extenders such as trisets and compound sets in a busy commercial gym, then you should adhere to a few simple rules:

1) **The fewer pieces of equipment the better**. If you can perform different exercises with the same piece of equipment, then that's ideal. Dumbbells and barbells work well in this regard. An example would be incline dumbbell curls followed immediately by standing dumbbell curls using the same weight.

2) **Have the equipment close by.** Again, free weights are ideal for this, because you can move them and position them right next to a machine that is stationary. An example would be pulldowns followed immediately by dumbbell pullovers performed over the seat of the pulldown station.

3) **Use bodyweight exercises when you can.** Bodyweight exercises such as pushups and sissy squats are ideal, because you can perform them at any time and without any equipment. You can easily and immediately follow-up a barbell or machine exercise with a bodyweight exercise. This minimizes the amount of equipment you need to set up, and it also minimizes the rest in between exercises. An example would be bench presses followed by pushups.

By sticking to these guidelines, you can stay at one or two stations and use one or two pieces of equipment rather than hog up multiple machine and stations and be interrupted by interlopers. You also minimize the rest in between exercises.

Key Points on Set Extenders:

- Set extenders allow you to extend the duration of muscular tension, which results in greater muscular growth.
- When constructing compound sets, pair exercises that complement each other and stress both sides of the muscle group.
- When constructing trisets, aggregate exercises that stress the entire strength curve.

Back Cycling:
Controlled Overtraining for Continuous Muscle Growth

VI. Back Cycling: Controlled Overtraining for Continuous Muscle Growth

In bodybuilding, change is good. Your body is highly adaptive, so developing a complete physique means you need variety: a variety of exercises, a variety of training programs.

Switching from program to program every so often is a good idea, but haphazardly switching programs just for the sake of switching doesn't always equate to progress. You're really just spinning your wheels. It's like going from job to job, but you're always working a minimum wage entry-level position.

Your body responds and grows better when you train hard for a while, then pull back. If you've been doing a program where you were busting your ass and training hard, then your next program needs to be simple and less intense. If you were training in a lackadaisical manner, then your next program should be one where you step it up a notch.

This strategy of two steps forward and one step back is known as "back cycling." Back cycling is when you purposely overtrain yourself for a short period of time and then pull back to allow your body to overcompensate with muscular growth.

Back cycling is not the same as "muscle confusion," which is simply a haphazard changing of routines without rhyme or reason. Back cycling is best described as "controlled overtraining."

Back cycling consists of 2 phases: a density phase and a deloading or "decompression" phase. In a density phase, you purposely increase the density of training for 2-3 weeks. In other words, you do will more work per unit of time. This means increased sets, reps, and exercises per workout, but the workout length will remain the same: 45-60 minutes. To pack in more sets, reps and exercises within this brief time frame, you must employ shorter rest periods and use set extenders as well. Think of it as putting your body into overdrive.

You cannot stay in overdrive forever, though. You have to pull back or "back cycle." Rather than focus on training density, you lower the volume and focus on training *intensity*. This means heavier weight, lower reps, higher rest periods and fewer sets and exercises. There are three popular approaches to back cycling:

1. Cutting back on training volume
2. Decompression of training frequency
3. Abbreviation of your exercise routine

1. Cutting Back on Training Volume

In this method of back cycling, you train with a high number of sets and reps for 2-3 weeks and then cut the volume down by at least 40-50% for 2-3 weeks.

An easy way to figure out how to back cycle using this method is to add up all the reps for each body part in a workout. If the rep totals are high, then switch to lower rep totals in your next program. If your totals are low, then switch to a program with a higher rep total.

The following is a series of popular set and rep schemes strung together in way to take advantage of this particular back cycling strategy:

Weeks	Sets	Reps	Rest	Total Volume
1, 2	10	10	1:00	100
3, 4	6	6	2:00	36
5, 6	8	8	0:30	64
7, 8	5	5	3:00	25
9, 10	4	12	1:30	48
11, 12	8	3	1:00	24

The sets and reps are for each body part that you wish to train. In order words, 10x10 means 10 sets of 10 reps for the chest, 10 sets of 10 reps for the back, and so on and so on.

Stay with each set and rep scheme for 2-3 weeks and then move on to the next. How you want to split the body parts and what split routine you want to use is up to you. Just don't go beyond 20 sets per workout.

2. Decompression of Training Frequency

In this method of back cycling, you'll train at a very high frequency for 1-2 weeks and then train at a low frequency for 2-3 weeks. This type of back cycling works well for body part specializations. In other words, if you wanted to devote a few weeks to bringing up a muscle group lagging in size or strength, then back cycling your training frequency is an effective strategy.

Let's say you've got a decent amount of muscle everywhere except for your calves. You can develop a two-phase program for the calves. For the first 2 weeks you train the calves 6 days a week. Then the following 3 weeks you reduce the volume to 3 days a week, every other day:

Saturday	Sunday	Monday	Tuesday	Wednesday	Thursday	Friday
Workout A	Workout B	Workout A	Workout B	Workout A	Workout B	*Off*
Workout A	Workout B	Workout A	Workout B	Workout A	Workout B	*Off*
Workout C	*Off*	Workout C	*Off*	Workout C	*Off*	*Off*
Workout C	*Off*	Workout C	*Off*	Workout C	*Off*	*Off*
Workout C	*Off*	Workout C	*Off*	Workout C	*Off*	*Off*

<u>Weeks 1, 2</u>

Alternate between Workouts A and B six days a week:

<u>Workout A</u>

A) **Standing one-legged calf raises (bodyweight only):** With this exercise, you will perform bodyweight-only one-legged calf raises off the edge of a calf block. One hand will be holding on to a stable support. Alternate between the left and right leg with little or no rest until you reach 100 reps on each calf. Start off a high number of reps at first, and then when your reps start falling below 10, rest for about 30 seconds and resume.
B) **Maintenance mode for all other body parts:** 3 sets of 6-8 reps for each muscle group.

<u>Workout B</u>

A) **Standing Machine Calf Raises:** 5 sets of 10-12 reps
B) **Leg press calf raises:** 3 sets of 20 reps
C) **Seated calf raises:** 2 sets of 25 reps

<u>Week 3-5</u>

Follow this workout three days a week, every other day:

<u>Workout C</u>

A) **Dumbbell Calf Raises:** 5 sets of 10-12 reps
B) **Seated calf raises:** 3 sets of 20 reps
C) **Maintenance mode for all other body parts:** 3 sets of 6-8 reps for each muscle group.

3. Abbreviated Exercise Routines

Here's a situation that plays itself out every so often in the gym: a frustrated skinny bastard follows a routine found in a muscle mag. The routine includes multiple exercises for each body part, as well as the kitchen sink. The skinny bastard follows the routine for a while and makes some initial progress, but then he plateaus and eventually burns out from the sheer volume of 20 sets per muscle group.

A strength enthusiast tells our skinny bastard to cut out the excess exercises and stick to heavy weight on basic compound movements and VOILA! Muscle growth!

Sound familiar?

Switching from multi-angular training to an abbreviated strength program is a form of back cycling. From a bodybuilding perspective, you must train a muscle group from more than one angle in order to fully maximize its size.

Yet from a strength perspective, there is little benefit to performing more than one exercise for a muscle group. Your nervous system gets confused performing so many different exercises. You will make the most progress in the first exercise targeting a muscle group, but you will not develop as much strength in succeeding exercises.

Alternating phases of bodybuilding-based training and powerlifting-based training allows you to develop both muscle symmetry and muscle mass. Here's a two-phased program that alternates typical bodybuilding-style training with an abbreviated strength program:

Rotate through the following three workouts. This is 3 day on/1 day off program. Rest periods are 60-90 seconds.

Workout A

Chest
Bench press – 5 sets, 8-10 reps
Incline dumbbell press – 5 sets, 8-10 reps
Pec deck flyes – 4 sets, 10-12 reps

Back
Lat pulldowns – 5 sets, 10-12 reps
Dumbbell rows – 4 sets, 8-10 reps
Seated cable rows – 4 sets, 8-10 reps

Workout B

Thighs
Barbell back squats – 4 sets, 10-12 reps
Leg press – 4 sets, 10-12 reps
Leg extensions – 4 sets, 10-12 reps
Leg curls – 4 sets, 6-8 reps

Calves
Standing machine calf raises – 4 sets, 15-20 reps
Donkey calf raises – 4 sets, 15-20 reps
Seated machine calf raises – 4 sets, 15-20 reps

Workout C

Shoulders
Military press – 5 sets, 8-10 reps
Laterals – 5 sets, 10-12 reps
Bent over laterals – 4 sets, 10-12 reps

Biceps
Barbell curls – 4 sets, 8-10 reps
Incline dumbbell curls – 4 sets, 10-12 reps
Preacher curls – 4 sets, 8-10 reps

Triceps
Lying triceps extensions – 4 sets, 6-8 reps
Overhead cable triceps extensions – 4 sets, 10-12 reps
Close grip barbell press – 4 sets, 8-10 reps

Weeks 3-6

Alternate between the following two workouts three days a week, every other day with weekends off:

Workout A

A) Bench Press - 6 sets of 3-6 reps, 3 minute rest periods
B) Deadlifts – 6 sets of 3-6 reps, 3 minute rest periods

Workout B

A) Pull-ups - 6 sets of as many reps as possible, 3 minute rest periods
B) Back Squats - 6 sets of 3-6 reps, 3 minute rest periods

Key Points on Back Cycling:

- Back cycling is purposely overtraining for a short period of time (density phase), then pulling back to allow your body to overcompensate with muscular growth (decompression phase).

- Three popular approaches to back cycling are:
  1. Cutting back on training volume
  2. Decompression of training frequency
  3. Abbreviation of your exercise routine

Quad Quest

VII. Quad Quest

While most bodybuilding newbies are motivated to pump up their upper bodies, the true hardcore lifter (and masochist) looks forward to blasting his thighs. Want to know who's a hardcore lifter? Does he squat a Mack truck, ass to the grass? Or is he doing lunges off a stability ball? This is when you know if he's got balls of steel and a cobra snake necktie or if he's into strength training (if you can call it strength training) for "metrosexual" reasons (not that there is anything wrong with that).

The question for you is: do you want to *be* strong and powerful or do you want your quads to *look* strong and powerful? Well, guess what? You can have both! It comes at the high price of muscle soreness, but hey, you were willing to pay that price anyway when you got that gym membership, right?

Choosing the Right Exercises

When most guys lift for quad size and/or tone, they usually pick these four exercises: back squats, leg presses, lunges and leg extensions. While these exercises can produce size and tone in the thighs overall, the size and tone produced by these exercises (with the exception of leg extensions) is not in the quadriceps. You'll get a big butt and some sore hamstrings if you squat all the way down, but the front of your thighs, the quadriceps, will remain under stimulated and underdeveloped.

Why concentrate on developing your quadriceps? If you look at an anatomy chart, you'll find that the lines separating your quadriceps muscles are vertical. If you create muscle separation between the quadriceps muscles and develop the vastus medialis in particular, then those vertical lines will make your thighs look powerful, yet long and sleek. The vastus medialis is the tear drop quad muscle above your knees, and it is the pivot point muscle that you want to build and emphasize for symmetry.

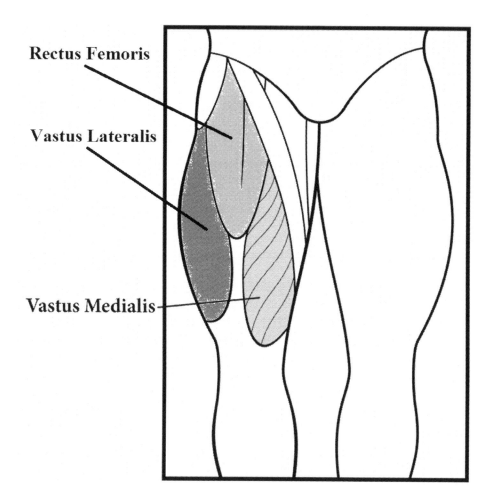

Rectus Femoris

Vastus Lateralis

Vastus Medialis

Back squats, leg presses and lunges stress the quads somewhat, but they primarily stress the glutes, hips, inner thighs and hamstrings. Bodybuilders desire hamstring size, and I discuss hamstring development in another chapter.

The development of the glutes, hips, and inner thighs, however, will widen your thighs and make you look short and stocky. If you want to build the vastus medialis and develop the long powerful look of your quads, then you'll have to rethink your exercises.

Squat Variations

Most people don't even squat in the first place, and when they do they only squat till their thighs are parallel. Yet if you want big powerful thighs and a big powerful physique in general, then you need to do full range squats (any squats), PERIOD.

But for quad emphasis, which squat variation do you choose? Front squats or back squats?

The thing with back squats is that they will hit your hamstrings, hips and glutes a lot harder than your quadriceps. Don't believe me? Do a couple of heavy sets of full range 20 rep breathing back squats and tell me the next day where you feel sore.

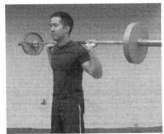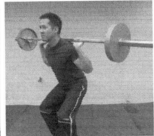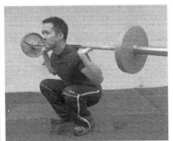

Back squat

That's right: you're sore in the hamstrings and sore in the ass (insert homo-erotic joke here). What about your quads? Any soreness? Unless that was your first time doing squats, then your answer would be a big, "NO!"

The **front squat**, however, hits your quadriceps much harder than back squats. When you do back squats, the bar is on you back, so you have to lean forward at the bottom to support and push the weight back up. Leaning forward activates the glutes and leaves your quads out of the action.

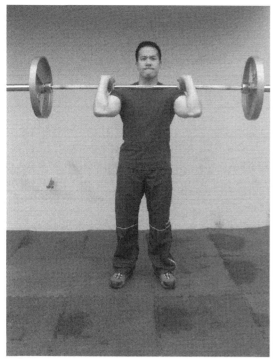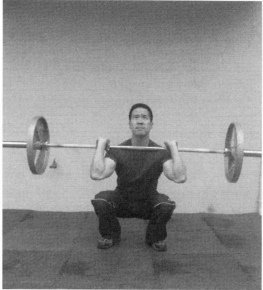

The Front Squat

The front squat does the exact opposite. Since the bar is in front of your body, you have to support the weight in an upright position. If you so much as lean forward, then you'll lose control of the barbell and you'll have crushed knees. Squatting in this upright position will activate your quads and your abdominals, leaving your glutes out of the picture. Instead of building up a big ass, you build up the long vertical lines of the quadriceps just above the knees.

People who dare to squat usually back squat, because they can lift more weight and the exercise is not as technically demanding. If you simply need to add mass to your thighs and don't care how that mass looks, then the back squat is a surefire way to add that mass.

The front squat, however, is more physically and mentally demanding, but far more rewarding for your physique. It is a man maker, because you must hold and lift the weight with your whole entire body, not just your legs.

Another squat variation that's a quad builder is the **Hack squat**. Although the machine variation is OK, the barbell Hack squat stresses not only the vastus medialis, but the entire body. It is like performing a deadlift, but with the bar behind your back.

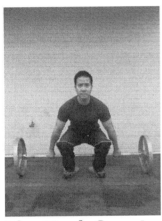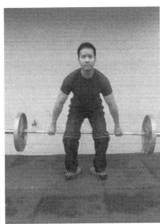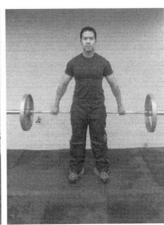

The Hack Squat

Sissy squats are another variation that stress the vastus medialis muscle but minimizes glute development. It is a deceptively simple exercise to perform, but it will reveal to you just how strong you are at the knees. Bend at the knees and lower yourself under control. Don't bend at the waist at any point during the exercise.

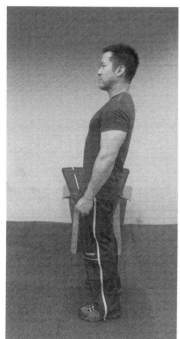 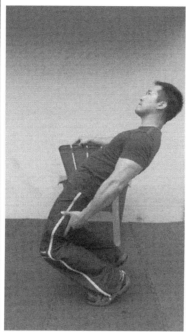 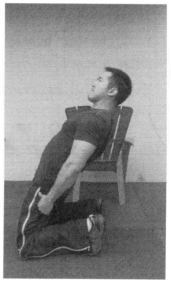

The Sissy Squat

Most people find it difficult to perform just with bodyweight. If you're a badass and can perform more than 15 reps in strict form, then hold a 25 to 45 pound plate in front of you for added resistance.

Single Leg Exercises

Single leg exercises require your quads to work much harder than they normally do, since you normally stand, walk or run on two legs. In other words, your left and right legs are accustomed to sharing the load between the two of them. Adding a single leg exercise to your program will overload your quads more than they're used to. Single leg exercises can give you newfound growth in the quads.

A lot of people do forward lunges for their single leg exercise. Forward lunges primarily stress the inner thighs and glutes, but don't build up the quads. Some experts say you can shorten the stride of the lunge to develop the quads, but even then I have never found forward lunges to be an effective quad builder.

There is a lunge variation that builds the quads and that is the **reverse lunge**. Instead of stepping forward with one leg, you step backward with one leg.

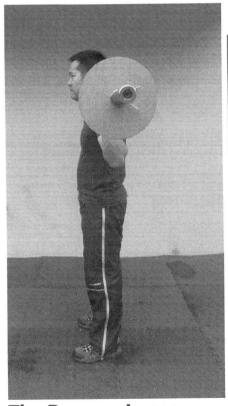 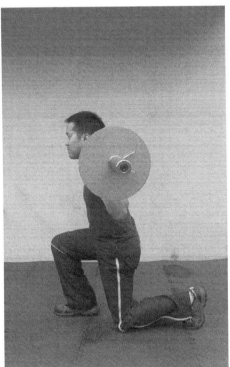

The Reverse Lunge

All lunges regardless of stride length stress the glutes, and the reverse lunge is no exception. Unlike the forward lunge, however, the reverse lunge also hits the outer quads (the vastus lateralis and rectus femoris) as well as the glutes. The reverse lunge will hit the outer quads harder than any squat variation.

Another single leg exercise is the **one-legged squat**, also known as the "Pistol." These require a lot of practice and flexibility, but once you're able to do them, pistols will leave you quite sore in the quads.

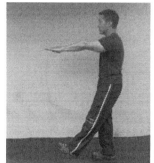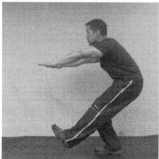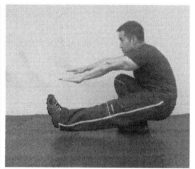

Pistols

To perform pistols, lower yourself on one leg while extending the other leg out in front of you. Sounds easy enough, right? If you don't concentrate, however, then you'll fall on your ass. Keep these points in mind when performing pistols:

- If you've never done pistols before, then perform half reps over a bench. Over the course of several workouts, increase the depth of your squat.
- Instead of arching your back as you would with barbell squats, you should round your back so that your torso is over the knee of the leg doing the squatting. By curling your torso over your knee as you squat to the bottom, your center of gravity stays directly over your base, which is your foot. This will help you avoid tipping over.

- Extend your arms out in front of you to counterbalance your torso as you squat down. Eventually you will be able to perform a lot of pistols, so you will need to hold a weight in front of you. The weight will serve as a nice counterweight to keep you balanced as you squat up and down.

Set Extenders for Massive Quads

The quadriceps has a very broad rep continuum. You can use low reps, high reps and everything in between, and the quadriceps will grow. Powerlifters and Olympic weightlifters squat heavy, and they build impressive quads. Speed skaters and bicyclists train with extremely high volumes of work, and their quads are also huge.

Tom Platz, famous for his enormous legs, squatted with a wide variety of reps. But he was known to have regularly squatted with ultra-high reps: multiple sets of 20-30 plus reps!

The quads crave high tension for long durations. If you make them lift heavy for a lot of reps, then your quads will blow up. This is why 20-rep breathing squats will build up massive thighs.

Twenty rep breathing squats were popularized by Ironman editor Peary Rader in the early days of bodybuilding, and it is the one method that consistently produces results. People looking to produce size always come back to this method to jumpstart their gains. The popular book "Super Squats" by Randall Strossen renewed interest in the technique.

If you're not familiar with breathing squats, it's really simple in theory, BRUTAL in execution. Take a 10-15 rep max weight for the back squat (full range version) and perform 20 reps instead. What will happen is you'll get to the 10-15th rep, stand still with the bar on your back, breathe a few breathes, then do another rep, breathe a few deep breathes, then do another rep, and so on and so forth until you reach 20 reps.

What you're essentially doing is a form of rest-pause for squats, but a better version of it. Breathing squats induce *hypoxia* (breathlessness). This state of oxygen debt forces your body to produce more red blood cells. More red blood cells mean more carriers of your body's major anabolic hormone: testosterone.

You'll be producing more testosterone, because of the heavy squatting. Lift heavy for an extended set, and your body will produce growth hormone as well.

The problem with squatting with such high reps is that your stabilizer muscles will give out before your quads do. Back squatting is very tough on the lower back. While your quads can handle ultra-high reps of heavy weight, your lower back cannot.

To lift heavy for an extended period of time, you can use set extenders such as trisets for the quads. This allows you to squat with a heavy weight and then extend the set by performing a non-weight bearing bodyweight exercise:

Quad Triset, Option #1:

20 Rep Breathing Squats followed immediately by
Sissy Squats (as many reps as possible with body weight only) followed immediately by
Leg Extensions (10-12 reps)
Rest for 5-6 minutes
Repeat one more time

This triset will nauseate you more than any other workout you've tried in the past. You'll experience massive hypoxia, and you'll find out that the 5-6 minutes rest will go by rather quickly. You'll also find that you won't be able to walk right for days. You will, however, feel some nice results almost overnight. One note of caution: don't attempt this triset on a full stomach!

The other advantage of this triset is that you're working through three different force curves for the quads:

Back squats- Midrange emphasis
Sissy squats- Bottom range emphasis
Leg extensions- Top range emphasis

Don't start out with this triset immediately. Start out with the breathing squats and do them at most once a week. Once you can handle 20-rep breathing squats, add in the rest of the triset.

Now if you can't perform the above triset without blowing chunks, then give this triset a try instead. Don't be surprised if you can't walk up the stairs for a week:

Quad Triset, Option #2:

Barbell Reverse Lunges (8-10 reps) followed immediately by
Back Squats (as many reps as possible with the same weight you used for lunges) followed immediately by
Sissy Squats (as many reps as possible with body weight only)
Rest for 3 minutes
Repeat the entire process two more times

Key Points on Quad Development:

- Use squat variations that target the vastus medialis.
- Use single leg exercises to overload the quads more than they accustomed to.
- Use a wide variety of reps for the quads.

The following is a specialization program for developing powerful looking quads. Exercise substitutions can be made after Week #1, but adhere to the prescribed sets and reps. Follow the program for 2-3 weeks.

Quadriceps Specialization Program	

Workout #1
 	
Quad Triset:
  1) Back squats (20 reps)
  2) Sissy squats (as many reps as possible)
  3) Leg extensions (10-12 reps)
  • Perform 2 trisets
  • Rest 6 minutes between trisets
	Workout #2
	
	Reverse barbell lunges (3 sets, 10-12 reps, 90 seconds rest)
	
	Perform 3 sets of 6-8 reps with 90 seconds rest for each of the following:
	
	  • Calves
	  • Chest
	  • Back
	  • Deltoids
	  • Biceps
	  • Triceps

Workout #3
 	
Front squats or Hack squats:
  • 10 sets of 4-6 reps
  • Rest 3 minutes between sets
	Workout #4
	
	Perform 3 sets of 6-8 reps with 90 seconds rest for each of the following:
	
	  • Calves
	  • Chest
	  • Back
	  • Deltoids
	  • Biceps
	  • Triceps
	  • Abs

You can perform the sequence of workouts throughout the week in the following manner:

Option #1

Day 1 – Workout #1
Day 2 – off
Day 3 – Workout #2
Day 4 – off
Day 5 – Workout #3
Day 6 – Workout #4
Day 7 – off

Option #2

Day 1 – Workout #1
Day 2 – Workout #2
Day 3 – off
Day 4 – Workout #3
Day 5 – Workout #4
Day 6 – off
Day 7 – off

Steel-Cabled Hamstrings

VIII. Steel-Cabled Hamstrings

For beginning to intermediate bodybuilders, the hamstrings remain the "undiscovered country" of size and strength. Most bodybuilders have a natural tendency to seek out and explore various exercises and programs for their upper bodies and even for their quads. They discover that squats and deadlifts add size not only to the thighs, but to the upper body as well.

Yet when it comes to program design specifically for the hamstrings, most bodybuilders (even veterans) are clueless. What happens is that bodybuilders will take the lessons they learned for quad size (i.e. 20 rep breathing squats) and then apply these lessons to hamstring training (i.e. ultra-high rep leg curls).

Twenty rep breathing squats will blow up your thighs till you look like a frog, and leg curls are essential to a thigh-building program, but high rep leg curls are useless. Yet most bodybuilders rely on high rep leg curls as their sole hamstring builder. You end up getting a bunch of bodybuilders with half built thighs: swollen quads, flat hamstrings.

How do you build thick hamstrings that look like steel cables going down the back of your thighs? As always the answer lies in understanding exercise selection and fiber makeup of the hamstrings.

The hamstrings consist of three muscles: the biceps femoris (which is all fast-twitch muscle fiber), the semitendinosus and the semimembranosus (both of which have a mix of fast and slow-twitch muscle fibers). Hence hamstring exercises can be categorized into 2 parts:

1) Exercises for the biceps femoris and
2) Exercises for the semitendinosus and the semimembranosus.

Perform an exercise from each category, and you will obtain complete hamstring development.

The Biceps Femoris

Exercises which work the biceps femoris are primarily leg curls: standing leg curls, seated leg curls and lying leg curls. This is the one occasion where machines are superior to free weights in developing a muscle, because no free weight exercises activate the biceps femoris like machine leg curls.

Since the biceps femoris are composed primarily of fast-twitch muscle fiber, they are designed for power. If you train your hamstrings for power then they will gain size as well. Muscular power is a combination of speed and strength. So how do you train your hamstrings for power and size?

#1: **Go heavy!** The biceps femoris responds extremely well to heavy weight at lower reps. Three to six reps is all you need for leg curls. Anything more is just a waste of time.

#2: **Go heavy, but FAST!** What's power again?

Strength (heavy) + Speed (FAST!) = Power

Powerful hamstrings = BIG hamstrings

So it's important to choose a weight that is heavy, but is light enough to allow you to move the weight as fast as possible. Again, 3-6 reps are the target rep range for leg curls.

#3: **Go heavy (but fast) over and over and over again!** Because you're using low reps, you have to make up for the lack of volume by doing multiple sets. Not 3-5 sets. Six sets and beyond. Without the added volume, you will not get the added size.

So why do people fail to build massive hamstrings on leg curls? The reason, again, is that they employ high reps (8-15). They think because the leg curl is an isolation exercise that they should use high reps.

If you are looking to build thick hamstrings, then you as a bodybuilder need to get out of the "high rep/isolation exercise" mindset and employ multiple sets of low reps for leg curls. Instead of 3-4 sets of 12-15 reps for leg curls, try 8-10 sets of 3-5 reps.

The Semitendinosus and Semimembranosus

For the semitendinosus and semimembranosus, choose exercises that are variations of stiff-legged deadlifts. Variations include Romanian deadlifts and good mornings. Since the semitendinosus and semimembranosus have a mix of fast and slow-twitch muscle fibers, you can employ higher reps for these exercises. The range should be 6-12 reps.

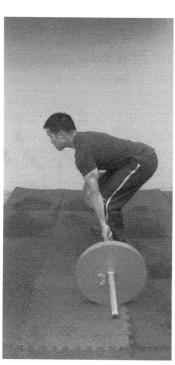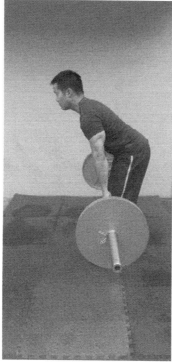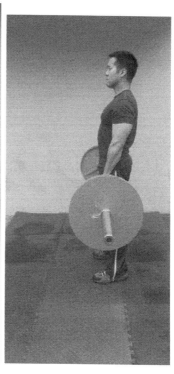

Romanian deadlifts:
- Keep the back straight
- Bend at the hips and lower your torso forward until it is parallel to the floor
- Keep the bar close to your legs as you lower it
- Allow for a slight bend at the knees and stick your butt back somewhat to take some of the stress off your lower back

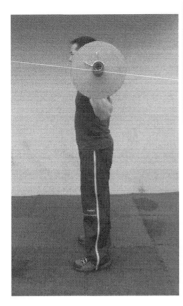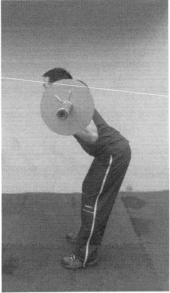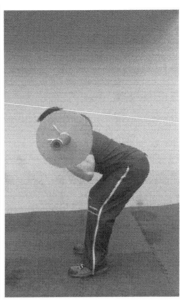

Good Mornings:
- Keep the back straight
- Bend at the hips and lower your torso forward until it is above parallel to the floor
- Allow for a slight bend at the knees to take some of the stress off your lower back

Although the semitendinosus and semimembranosus have a mix of fast and slow-twitch fibers, they will respond more favorably to lower reps and heavier weight over time. The more you train, the more your body will respond to lower reps and heavier weights. So while you may start out with 3 sets of10-12 reps on good mornings in your early phases of hamstring training, over time you'll be doing be 4 or more sets of 6-8 reps. As a bodybuilder, you will instinctively move towards lower reps, because you will find your hamstrings will grow bigger in response.

Building Thicker Hamstrings with Squats and Deadlifts

As mentioned in the Quad Quest chapter, full range back squats will build up the glutes and hamstrings. Even though your quads are the prime movers when you squat, your hamstrings have to isometrically contract to control your descent, particularly when you squat past parallel.

This is known as "Lombard's Paradox." Even though the quads and hamstrings are antagonistic muscles, both muscles will contract when you squat.

This is the reason why full range squats build bigger thighs than half squats. Squatting till your thighs are parallel with the floor will only work the quads. Squatting past parallel will work the quads and the hamstrings.

Lombard's Paradox also applies to deadlifts as well. Deadlifts will build strong, powerful hamstrings as well as a thick muscular back. The deadlift corrects many postural problems, but only if it is done properly. Many people fail to straighten out completely when performing the deadlift. At the top of each rep, you should straighten yourself out completely, sticking your chest out, keeping your shoulders down and squeezing your shoulder blades back.

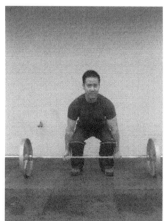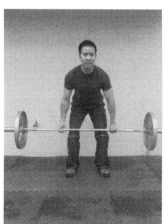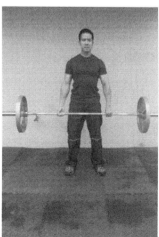

Deadlifts

Deadlifts do not build as much lower body mass as full range squats, but they are better at building muscle throughout your body overall. If you want to emphasize the glutes, hamstrings and quads more, then you can perform the sumo deadlift. The sumo version is also less taxing on the lower back. Simply take a wider stance and grasp the bar with a shoulder width grip.

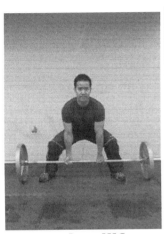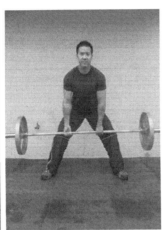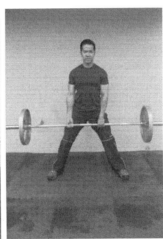

Sumo deadlifts

Remember the Mantra...

Go heavy. Go FAST! Over and over and over again. Do this, and your hamstrings will transform into bundles of steel cables.

Other key points on hamstring training:
- Use leg curls to develop the biceps femoris.
- Use stiff-legged deadlift variations to develop the semitendinosus and semimembranosus.
- Take advantage of Lombard's Paradox and do deadlifts and full range squats to build up your hamstrings.

The following is specialization program designed to increase the size and power of your hamstrings. Exercise substitutions can be made after Week #1, but follow the prescribed sets and reps. Follow the program for 2-3 weeks.

Hamstrings Specialization Program	
Workout #1 Back squats: • 6 sets of 6-8 reps • Rest 3 minutes between sets Lying leg curls: • 6 sets of 4-6 reps • Fast positive, slow negative • Rest 3 minutes between sets	**Workout #2** Romanian deadlifts (3 sets, 8-10 reps, 90 seconds rest) Perform 3 sets of 6-8 reps with 90 seconds rest for each of the following: • Calves • Chest • Back • Deltoids • Biceps • Triceps
Workout #3 Standing one-legged machine curls or Seated leg curls: • 10 sets of 3-5 reps • Fast positive, slow negative • Rest 3 minutes between sets	**Workout #4** Perform 3 sets of 6-8 reps with 90 seconds rest for each of the following: • Calves • Chest • Back • Deltoids • Biceps • Triceps • Abs

You can perform the sequence of workouts throughout the week in the following manner:

Option #1

Day 1 – Workout #1
Day 2 – off
Day 3 – Workout #2
Day 4 – off
Day 5 – Workout #3
Day 6 – Workout #4
Day 7 – off

Option #2

Day 1 – Workout #1
Day 2 – Workout #2
Day 3 – off
Day 4 – Workout #3
Day 5 – Workout #4
Day 6 – off
Day 7 – off

Wingspan Exercises

IX. Wingspan Exercises

Let's face it: people respect strength. People respond differently when you're built like an ox. When people can see *from your front* that your back is a mountain of muscle and that your forearms resemble bundles of steel cables, they realize this:

1) You're strong.
2) You've put in some hard work and hard time to become strong.
3) You're disciplined enough to do the hard work and the hard time to become strong.

These qualities (strength, hard work, discipline) earn you respect, regardless of your background. The cornerstone of this look that commands respect is a thick, wide, muscular back. While a wide V-tapered back is a sign of the classical bodybuilder, a V-tapered back that is also thick and muscular is a sign of a power bodybuilder, a lifter who values strength as well as aesthetics.

To build a thick V-tapered back, you should concentrate on three goals in your upper back training:

1. Back width characterized by a V-taper (wide at the shoulders, tapering as you go down)
2. Back thickness characterized by a muscular mid-back
3. Minimal trapezius development

A bodybuilder should avoid overdeveloping the upper trapezius muscle, since the downward slope of massive traps will detract from a V-taper and give you an A-taper instead. The trapezius will grow from ANY heavy standing barbell exercise (such as deadlifts and cleans), so it is not necessary to perform exercises which target the trapezius directly (such as shrugs and narrow grip upright rows).

A muscular V-taper back should be built primarily through pull-ups, chin-ups, deadlifts, cleans and rows. I differ from most strength trainers, because I don't recommend barbell rows for back development. This is not to say that the barbell row isn't an effective exercise. But when it comes to feeling your back during a workout and the day after, there really is no comparison between pull-ups and barbell rows.

A lot of bodybuilders choose barbell rows to develop back thickness. Barbell rows, however, suck big time as a back exercise, especially for the beginning lifter. The back muscles go through a limited range of motion when performing barbell rows.

Barbell rows don't stretch your lats, and it's hard to get a peak contraction of your back muscles at the top of the movement. Most people heave the weight up, which makes the tension at full contraction very brief and ineffective. If you slowed down the movement, then you'd have to use less weight, which would make the exercise even more ineffective.

What's more is when you perform the barbell row your neural drive is split between contracting your lower back and hamstrings and rowing the weight. In other words, your body has to do 2 different things at the same time. It's like juggling while riding a unicycle. You end up working a multitude of body parts and not very well. A great overall body exercise, but not a very good *back* exercise.

The following are 3 exercises that will forge major mountains and valleys in the musculature of your back without splitting up your nerve force. Instead of moving the weight *and* stabilizing your own body weight, you concentrate solely on moving the weight. If you're looking to thicken your back, then you should include some of these exercises in your program:

Deadlifts for Back Thickness

In addition to developing a thick back, the deadlift corrects many postural problems, but only if it is done properly. Many people fail to straighten out completely when performing the deadlift. Failure to straighten your back out completely will aggravate the hunched over caveman look. At the top of each rep, you should straighten your torso out, sticking your chest out and squeezing your shoulder blades back. This will engage your lower trapezius and rhomboids.

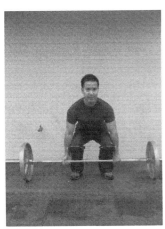 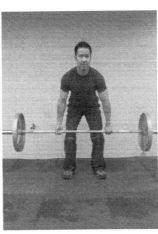 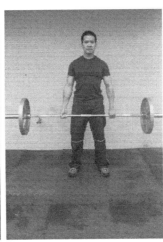

Wide grip deadlifts

Performing the deadlift with a wide grip will engage the back more so than regular deadlifts. This is a great exercise not just for the legs, but for your lats, since they must isometrically contract to hold the weight. If you don't know how to do a lat spread bodybuilding pose, then this harsh exercise will beat the snot out of you to teach you.

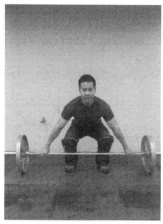 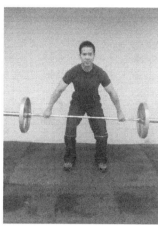 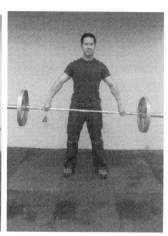

Power Cleans

Power cleans will not only develop a thick back, but explosiveness as well. To perform a power clean, stand over a barbell and grab it with an over hand grip slightly wider than shoulder width. Bend at the knees and hips and keep your lower back arched. Pull your body up so that the barbell touches mid-thigh.

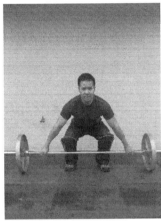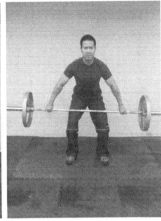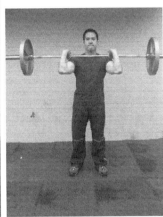

Jump up and extend your torso. Shrug at the shoulders and pull the barbell upward. This should be done explosively. As you pull the bar up, your body will drop underneath the bar, resting the weight on your shoulders.

Developing Back Width through Pull-ups

Rows, deadlifts and cleans are great for back thickness, but not for back width. Your lats don't get much of a stretch from rows, deadlifts or cleans. If you want a wingspan that would make an eagle envious, then you got to do pull-ups and chin-ups.

You can certainly do lat pulldowns to widen your back, but as far as developing both size and strength, pull-ups and chin-ups are superior to cable pulldowns. The reason is that there is more negative tension from pull-ups and chin-ups. With cable pulldowns (and with machines in general) there is very little negative tension since the weight is on a pulley system.

Most people, however, have a difficult time doing pull-ups. The pull-up is completely and utterly unforgiving. You either can do a pull-up, or you cannot. Your chin passes the finish line that is the bar, or you hang there helpless. That bar is a clear demarcation of manhood. So if you want to have a big badass back, then you better learn how to do some pull-ups.

What if you can't perform a pull-up, but you want to develop a thick wide back that busts doorframes every time you walk through them? If this is the case, then your goal in back training is two-fold:

1) Develop a massive back with a combination of free weights (deadlifts, elbows out dumbbell rows and pullovers) and cable exercises (pulldowns and short pulley rows).
2) Develop your vertical pulling strength by working on intermediary exercises for the pull-up.

If you cannot do a pull-up, then the following techniques will help you develop the lat strength to perform one (provided you are not overweight).

Increase Your Dead Hang Time

To perform pull-ups, then you have to stay on the bar long enough to perform the exercise. If you cannot last a minute hanging from a bar, then you should concentrate on increasing your dead hang time. Dead hang time is about isometric strength or holding yourself in a static position. There are 3 factors involved in dead hangs:

1) Dead Hang Form- The easiest way to hang is to let your arms and body hang straight down. Don't move or sway a lot. Just take a shoulder width grip. Anything wider than shoulder-width makes it harder on you. While hanging, make sure your shoulder blades are tight and retracted back. Your shoulders should be pulled in tight. Do not relax your shoulders and allow your body to sag further. Allowing this to happen will pull your shoulders out of their sockets.

2) Breathing and Contracting- You have to breathe in a slow and relaxed manner, but contract your upper body muscles. Make sure that you make each breathe last as long as you can. When you exhale, tighten your grip and your abs.

When you train to prolong your dead hang time, don't go to failure. Hang on the bar for as long as you can, but as soon as you feel your grip loosening, then it's time to stop. Rest for 10-20 seconds, and then get back on. Keep repeating until you can no longer hold yourself for even 10 seconds. Once you've reached that point, it's time to stop and end that exercise. Try to do this every day. Test your dead hang time once a week.

3) Grip Strength- If you're slipping off the bar because you cannot hold on any longer, then you should work on your isometric grip strength. Do some fat bar training if you have access to some thick bars. Barbells, dumbbells and kettlebells with thick handles will develop your grip strength and forearms, even when you're performing exercises meant to target other muscle groups.

Intermediary Pull-up Exercises

Once you can hang on a bar for over a minute with ease, then it's time to perform intermediary exercises that will build your strength and teach you to perform an actual pull-up:

Start with the easiest pull-up variation and do partial reps. If you can, then start out with pull-ups with a narrow and neutral grip. In other words, palms facing each other. This is the easiest form of pull-ups. If you do not have access to a pull-up station with a V-bar handle, then use a shoulder width underhand grip. Pull yourself up from a dead hang position as far as you can go. If this means half reps in the bottom position, then perform as many partial reps as you can short of failure.

Do some partner assisted pull-ups. This will teach your body how to do pull-ups, but you have to have a partner that gives you just the right amount of assistance. If he's heaving you up every time, and you're doing jack, then there's really no point. So make sure your partner gives you the minimal amount of assistance to help you with the pull-ups.

Don't do the machine-assisted pull-ups. Pull yourself up as far as you can go, then have your workout partner assist you the rest of the way up. Once you're up there with your chin above the bar, your partner will let go and YOU WILL HOLD THAT POSITION FOR AS LONG AS YOU CAN.

Once you can't hold that position at the top, lower yourself as slowly as possible. This will expose your back muscles to significant overload in the top range position, which is something your back muscles aren't getting if you only do partial pull-ups. Do this one set of one negative rep at the beginning of every workout.

Don't do machine assisted pull-ups, because it offers no real benefit to helping you learn how to do a pull-up. Do partner assisted pull-ups instead. Over time your partner should be applying less and less assistance in your pull-ups. Eventually you will perform an actual pull-up and an actual chin-up.

Perform negative pull-ups. You can perform negatives pull-ups without the help of a spotter: position an Olympic barbell on a squat rack or on a Smith machine just high enough for you to perform pull-ups with your knees bent. Grab on to the bar, fold your legs and lower yourself under control. Stand up and position your body back at the top of the pull-up movement. Fold your legs again and perform another negative rep. Try to complete 3 negative pull-ups.

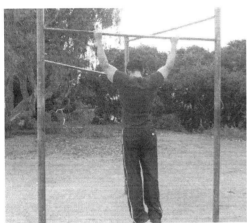 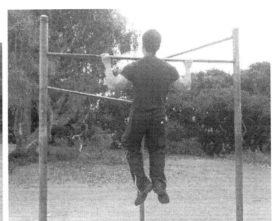

Pull-ups (overhand grip)

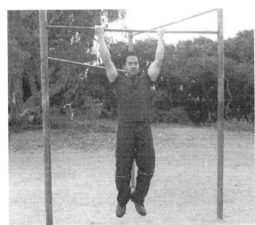 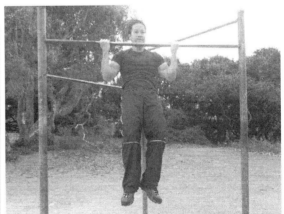

Chin-ups (underhand grip)

Using High Frequency Training to Increase Your Pull-ups

Once you can perform pull-ups and chin-ups, your goal then will be to increase the number of pull-ups and chin-ups. The best way to increase the number of pull-ups and chin-ups is to employ *high frequency training* (HFT). You can use HFT to increase your strength or reps on any exercise, as long as you choose only one exercise in which to improve your performance on.

The way HFT works is you perform one set of pull-ups at the beginning of every workout. So if you work out 4 times a week, then you will perform 4 sets of pull-ups for the entire week. At minimum you must work out three times spread over the course of a week. Ideally you should perform one set of pull-ups 4-6 times per week.

DO NOT GO TO FAILURE when performing pull-ups on the HFT program. If you start doing half reps, or if the speed of your reps slows down (like you're stuck in mid rep), then you know you are reaching muscular failure and you should stop the set right then and there.

When you can perform at least 10 reps controlled full range pull-ups, then you should add a second set. In other words, do 2 sets of pull-ups or chin-ups before every workout. You'll rest for 3 minutes in between the 2 sets. Again, do not go to muscular failure on either set.

Once you can perform 2 sets of 10-12 full range pull-ups, you can add weight by attaching a plate or dumbbell on a weight belt. Adding weight will not only increase your pull-up strength, but it will also increase your strength endurance. It seems counterintuitive, but if you strap on weight and focus on low reps (4-6), then you'll increase your repetitions when you go back to simple bodyweight only pull-ups.

Pull-up Variations

You should also expand your pull-up repertoire and start performing more difficult pull-up and chin-up variations:

Mixed grip chin-ups- This exercise is the precursor to the one handed chin-up. Not only will this exercise work the lats, but it will overload the biceps more than they're used to.

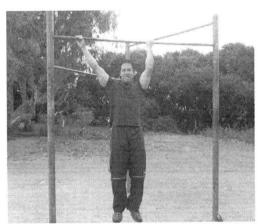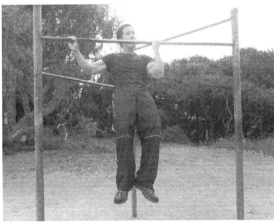

With this exercise you perform a chin-up with one hand supinated (underhand grip) and one hand farther out on the bar pronated (overhand grip). The side with the underhanded grip takes on more of the load. Be sure to perform an equal amount of reps for both sides. If you're weaker on one side, then start with the weaker arm in the supinated position.

Side to side pull-ups- Once you get the hang (no pun intended) of regular wide grip pull-ups, then give this one a shot. This variation is analogous to performing alternating dumbbell curls, but with pull-ups. To perform this exercise, assume a wide-grip pull-up position by placing the hands a little wider than the shoulders. Instead of pulling yourself straight up to the bar, pull yourself towards one hand, alternating from side to side.

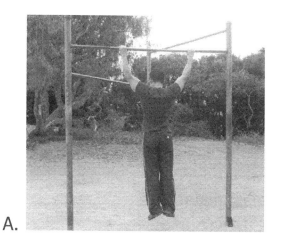

A.

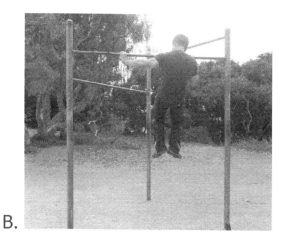

B.

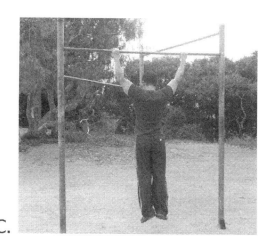

C.

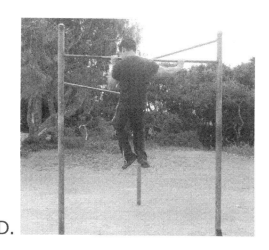

D.

The Sternum Chin-up- If pull-ups are the king of back exercises, then the sternum chin-up is the king of kings. Whereas conventional pull-ups develop the lats and teres major, sternum chin-ups provide complete back development by developing the lats, teres major and midback.

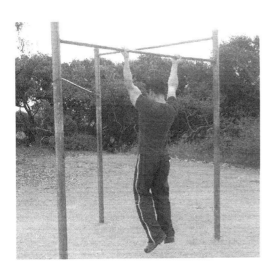 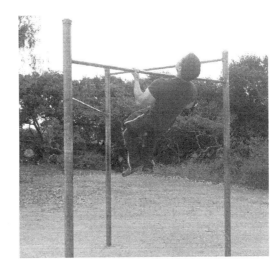

To perform the sternum chin-up, use an underhand grip slightly wider than your shoulders. Pull yourself up to the bar, extend your head as far back as possible and arch your spine. Keep pulling until your collarbone passes the bar and your sternum touches it. At the end of the movement, your head should be parallel to the floor and your hips and legs will be at a 45-degree angle to the floor.

The Subscapularis Pull-up- If you think sternum pull-ups are tough, then this pull-up variation will beat the snot out of you. This pull-up variation will give you complete upper back development, giving you both width and thickness. The subscapularis pull-up will work the lats, the teres major and the rhomboids.

Take a wide overhand grip and pull yourself up until the upper pecs touch the chin-up bar. This concentric portion of the movement is performed just like a regular pull-up.

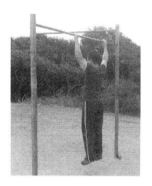 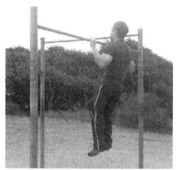 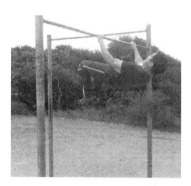

Once you get to this top position, however, you will push yourself *away* from the bar, lowering yourself under control. To help you perform this eccentric portion of the movement, pretend you are using the chin-up bar to do a bench press in mid-air. As you're pressing against the bar, your lats should be flexed and your shoulder blades squeezed back.

Target the Teres Major for a V-Taper

Most people assume building a V-tapered back means simply widening the lats. But this is not entirely true. Overdeveloped lats can detract from a bodybuilder's V-taper. Instead of a V-taper, overdeveloped lats coupled with overdeveloped traps will give you a diamond shaped back: ◇

You should build up the lats to some degree, but to develop width across your upper back you will need to focus on building up the **teres major**. The teres major is a pivot point muscle located under your armpit, in between your posterior deltoid and latissimus dorsi. When people talk about developing their "high lats" or upper lat area, they're really talking about developing their teres major muscles. The teres major is sometimes referred to as the "Little Lat" since it assists the lats in pulling and rowing exercises.

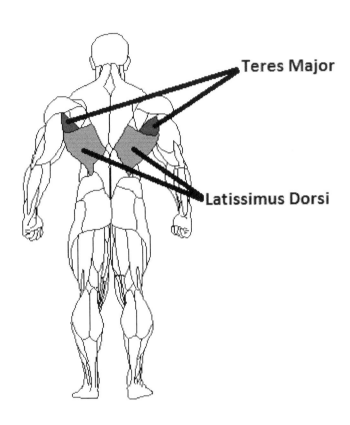

Although the teres major assists in all pulling and rowing exercises, the Little Lat is underdeveloped in most bodybuilders. The reason is that for many back exercises, the lats will do most of the work and leave the "Little Lat" with very little mechanical tension to grow on. Hence many bodybuilders have overdeveloped lats and underdeveloped teres major muscles. They lack width on top at the shoulder level.

The key to developing the teres major is to supplement your back program with exercises that specifically target the teres major but don't stress the lats. This is hard to do since you can't fully isolate a muscle. Muscles like to work together, and the big brother lats will always be there to back up the teres major.

An exercise that targets the teres major is the elbows out dumbbell row:

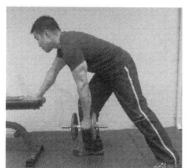 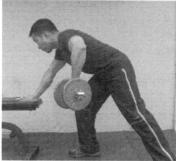 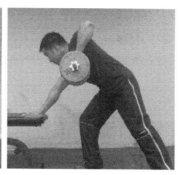

Elbows out dumbbell rows:
- Lean over the end of a bench and place one arm on it.
- The opposite leg should be positioned back.
- With your free hand grab a dumbbell from the floor and pull it towards you.
- Instead of pulling the dumbbell to the side of your ribs, pull with your elbow out to the side, away from your torso.
- At the top of the movement, your upper arm should be horizontally aligned with your shoulders and lower trapezius.
- Since the teres major is composed primarily of slow-twitch muscle fiber, shoot for a target rep range of 10-12 reps, fast positive/fast negative.

<u>Set Extenders for the Back</u>

If you've never felt your lats fully flexed, then you will definitely feel it with the triset listed below. This triset will hit the entire strength curve: midrange, stretch, contracted.

Only advanced bodybuilders should perform this technique. DO NOT even think about attempting this triset until you've learned how to perform the exercises properly by themselves:

> a) **Pulldowns** (8-10 reps) followed immediately by
> b) **Dumbbell pullovers** (8-10 reps) followed immediately by
> c) **Stiff-arm pulldowns** (8-10 reps)
> d) Rest 3-4 minutes
> e) Repeat 2 more times

Make sure you get a good stretch on the pullovers and flex the lats real hard on the stiff-arm pulldowns. If you're working out at home, and you don't have a cable machine, then you can substitute pull-ups for the pulldowns and barbell rows for the stiff-arm pulldowns. For these barbell rows, however, you should use an underhand grip on an EZ-curl bar.

If you can do pull-ups, then here's a giant set of pull-up variations that will blast every fiber in your back:

Wide-grip pull-ups (overhand grip) to failure. Rest 10 seconds.
Medium-grip pull-ups to failure. Rest 10 seconds.
Medium-grip chin-ups (underhand grip) to failure. Rest 10 seconds.
Narrow-grip chin-ups to failure.
Rest 3-4 minutes, then repeat the entire process 2 more times.

Key Points on Back Training:

- For strength and size, choose pull-ups and chin-ups over pulldowns.
- Target the teres major and avoid targeting the trapezius directly.
- Develop back thickness through deadlifts and cleans.

The following is specialization program designed to give your back a V-taper. Exercise substitutions can be made after Week #1, but follow the prescribed sets and reps. Follow the program for 2-3 weeks.

Back Specialization Program	

Workout #1
 	
Back Triset:
   1) Pulldowns (10-12 reps)
   2) Dumbbell pullovers (6-8 reps)
   3) Stiff-arm pulldowns (8-10 reps)
  • Perform 3 trisets
  • Rest 4 minutes between trisets
	Workout #2
	
	Elbows out dumbbell rows (3 sets, 10-12 reps, 90 seconds rest)
	
	Perform 3 sets of 6-8 reps with 90 seconds rest on the following:
	
	• Quadriceps
	• Hamstrings
	• Calves
	• Chest
	• Deltoids
	• Triceps

Workout #3 Pull-ups or Chin-ups: • Choose a variation of the pull-up • Perform 10 sets • Perform as many reps as possible on each set • Do not train to muscular failure • Rest for 3 minutes between sets	**Workout #4** Perform 3 sets of 6-8 reps with 90 seconds rest on the following: • Quadriceps • Hamstrings • Calves • Chest • Deltoids • Triceps • Abs

You can perform the sequence of workouts throughout the week in the following manner:

Option #1

Day 1 – Workout #1
Day 2 – off
Day 3 – Workout #2
Day 4 – off
Day 5 – Workout #3
Day 6 – Workout #4
Day 7 – off

Option #2

Day 1 – Workout #1
Day 2 – Workout #2
Day 3 – off
Day 4 – Workout #3
Day 5 – Workout #4
Day 6 – off
Day 7 – off

Forging the Armor-Plated Chest

X. Forging the Armor-Plated Chest

The chest is, arguably, the muscle most loved by bodybuilders. Aside from the arms, no other body part is given as much attention in the gym. Most newbies overemphasize the importance of the bench press and the pectoral muscles in their training programs. They put the bench press first in their workouts. They focus on getting stronger on this particular lift, because everybody asks, "How much you bench?" as if the bench press is an accurate indicator of real world strength.

With all this emphasis on chest training, people tend to fixate on chest size as opposed to chest shape. An overdeveloped chest can detract from muscle symmetry. An overdeveloped chest will give you 2 things:

1. Man-boobs
2. Poor posture

In other words, you'll look like a Neanderthal woman!

What you want to do is give your pecs a more angular look. You want to develop just enough thickness in the chest so that there's a horizontal shadow line below your lower pecs. This shadow line should go up the outer edges of your pecs and feed into your deltoids.

Instead of man-boobs (_|_) you want a wide tapering chest which resembles armor _|_/.

Here are the best exercises for the chest that I've come across in all my years of training. These exercises will develop thickness in the upper and lower pectorals. They will also give your chest the armor-plated look. This isn't the usual "bench press, incline press, dumbbell press, dumbbell flye" list for the chest, so do pay attention to the directions outlined in this chapter:

1) Gironda dips

This version of the dip is named after Vince Gironda, the Iron Guru who first came up with the idea to perform dips in this manner. It is the single best for the lower pectorals, hands downs! It's an excruciatingly difficult exercise to perform at first, but no other chest exercise is going to give you such immediate results.

To perform this exercise, you need a V-bar dipping station. Instead of gripping the bars with your palms facing each other (the way you would in regular dips), place your hands on the bars so that your palms facing away from each other. In this position, your elbows will stick out to the sides, which is what they should be doing throughout the exercise.

With your fingers and thumbs on the inside of these bars, perform the dips with your body shaped liked a crescent moon. In other words round out your back (don't arch it!), keep your chest in a concave position, and keep your feet forward in front of you. Be sure you dip all the way down to really stretch those pecs. You're going to feel incredibly sore for a few days, but you'll definitely notice a thickness to your lower chest that wasn't there before.

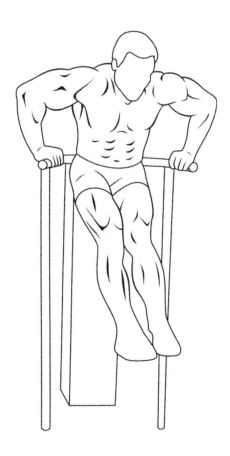

After just a few sets of this exercise, you'll wonder why your lower pecs never got this pumped before. If you have any issues with shoulder pain, however, then do not perform this exercise.

This exercise will thicken your lower pecs as well as the outer edges that connect to your shoulders. It will give you an armor plated chest that is tapered _|_/ as opposed to the man-boobs that you normally see on an overdeveloped chest (_|_).

2) Bench Press/Pushup compound set

Bodybuilders don't normally think of pushups as a mass builder for the chest. We usually of the bench press as the cornerstone exercise for pec size. Pushups as a set extender, however, will bring added mass and density to those pecs.

Here's what you do: perform any pressing movement for the chest. It could be the bench press, dumbbell incline press, or any other pressing movement. After you've gone to failure on that exercise and racked the bar (or dropped the dumbbells), immediately perform as many pushups as you can.

Although it is not necessary, you can perform these pushups while gripping a pair of dumbbells on the floor. Performing pushups on a pair of dumbbells will stretch your pecs provided that you descend all the way down. The dumbbells should be positioned wide enough to give you the same grip as on the bench press. If you want to stress the upper pecs more on the pushups, then perform them with your feet up on the bench.

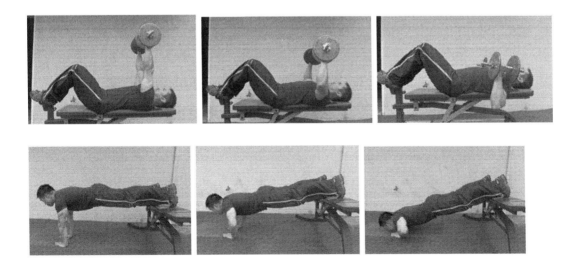

A few of these compound sets and you'll stroll around the gym looking like an armored tank!

3) The Neck Press (a.k.a. the Guillotine Press)

It looks like the bench press, but with one important difference: you lower the bar as close to your clavicles as you possibly can. When most weightlifters perform the bench press, they tend to lower the bar down on their nipples.

While this may be the best way to lift the most weight on the bench press, the Guillotine press is a far superior mass-builder than the conventional bench press. By simply lowering the bar to your neck and clavicle area and keeping your elbows as far from your torso as possible, you give your pectorals a greater stretch, which induces greater muscle growth.

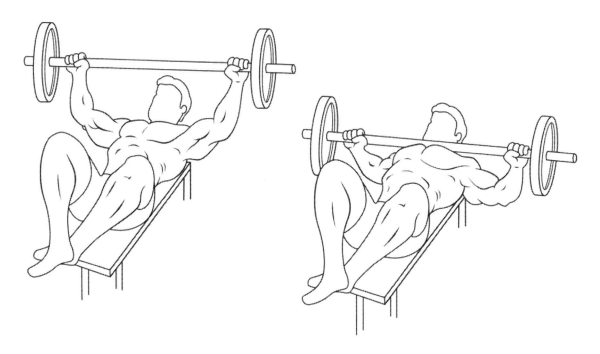

Like Gironda dips, however, there are couple things you should note:

a. When performing the Guillotine press, you should use less weight than you would normally use on the conventional bench press. Experiment first with lighter weight, then add more weight when you feel comfortable.

b. Don't perform this movement if you have shoulder problems.

4) The 20° Incline Press

This movement should be self-explanatory. By performing dumbbell presses or barbell presses on a 20-30° incline, you'll target the upper pecs. The problem, however, is that most incline benches are far too steep (they're usually at 45°). Performing incline presses at such a steep angle will stress more of your frontal deltoids and very little of your upper pecs. In fact, MRI studies show that decline presses will hit your upper pecs just as much as the 45° incline press.

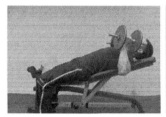 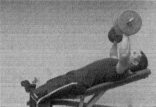 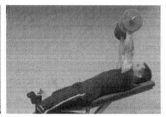

If your gym doesn't have any 20-30° incline benches, then don't worry about it. If you want to emphasize your upper pecs on a 45° incline bench, then use a narrower grip (about shoulder width). Guillotine presses and pushups with your feet elevated will also hit your upper pecs.

5) Dumbbell Presses

Mature bodybuilders instinctively know that for virtually all upper body exercises involving free weights, dumbbell movements are superior to their barbell counterparts in stimulating mass. For example, dumbbell bench presses pack more meat on your pecs than barbell bench presses.

The reason dumbbell movements tend to be superior to barbell movements has to do with neuromuscular stimulation. The greater the balance and coordination needed to move a weight, the greater the neuromuscular stimulation. When you lift dumbbells, more muscle fibers are recruited to perform the movement. Greater fiber recruitment translates to greater growth.

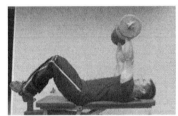 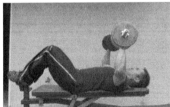 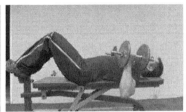

6) Machine Flyes

I may be in the minority, but when it comes to stretch-induced growth in the pectorals, I think machine flyes are superior to dumbbell flyes (provided that you're using the right machine). If you're using one of those padded pec deck machines where you're performing a shoulder adduction with the arms externally rotated (in other words, each of your arms is L-shaped as if you're in the middle of performing a military press), then you could incur long term damage to your shoulder joints.

Instead, use a pec deck with a pair of handles for you to grip rather than a couple of pads. This type of machine more closely resembles the movement of dumbbell flyes, which is much safer.

I like performing machine flyes instead of dumbbell flyes for a couple of reasons. With dumbbell flyes, all you feel is a stretch at the bottom third of the movement, but you don't feel any tension when you bring the dumbbells together.

But with machine flyes, there's constant tension on your pecs throughout the range of motion. Thus, not only do you get a good stretch at the beginning of each concentric rep, but you also fully contract your chest at the end of each concentric rep (unlike dumbbell flyes or the bench press).

The other reason that machine flyes are better than dumbbell flyes is that negatives are much more effective on a pec deck. Give this a try: after several sets on the bench press, finish off your chest workout with a few sets of machine flyes.

For each set on the pec deck, select a weight that will allow you to perform 10-12 reps in a quick tempo fashion. After you go to failure somewhere between the 10th and 12th rep, immediately perform 3 negatives with the next highest weight.

Make sure that with each rep, you fight the force of the weight until you're stretching back as far as you can go. Have a partner assist you in bringing the handles of the machine back to the beginning of each negative rep.

You shouldn't perform these eccentric sets all the time; just once every 2 weeks. Periodically performing negatives on the deck, however, will definitely provide you with consistent gains in chest size.

7) Side to Side Pushups

Although regular pushups are a great way to flush the chest and triceps muscles with blood, high rep pushups alone don't add much muscle. Most men over time can perform well over 20 pushups. Although you may get a great burn from high rep sets of pushups, they don't produce much muscular tension, because the weight is so low. You're only pressing, at most, half your bodyweight.

One-arm pushups are a great way to high muscular tension, but instead of stressing the chest, the tension shifts heavily to your triceps, lats, abs and legs. Plus most people find the one-arm pushup difficult to do.

A moderately difficult pushup that produces high tension in the chest is the "side to side pushup," also known as a "typewriter pushup." The side to side pushup produces high muscular tension in the chest, because most of the movement is performed in the bottom range. The pectoral muscles are only stressed in the bottom range of any bench press or pushup, so the side to side pushup is ideal for stressing the pecs.

To perform the side to side pushup, get into a starting pushup position.

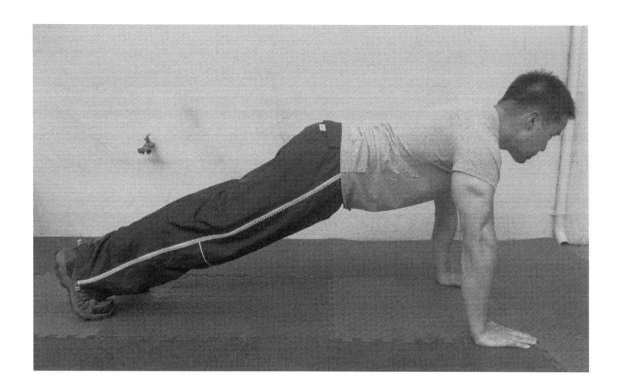

- Instead of lowering yourself straight down, you will lower yourself to one side. So if you choose to start with your left side, lower yourself to your left hand.
- Once you're at this bottom position, glide your body over to your right hand without letting your torso touch the ground.
- Push up from the right hand. That's one rep.
- Reverse the sequence of movements. This time you will lower yourself to your right hand, glide your body to your left hand and push up. That's two reps.
- Repeat until failure.

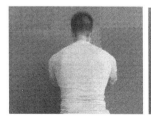 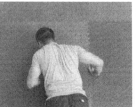 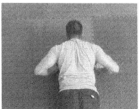 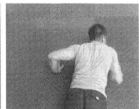

Chest Specialization Program

As you can see from this list, stretching, tension, and angle of execution are the three most important factors in training for chest size and more importantly chest shape. Make sure you incorporate these factors in your chest program regardless of what exercises you perform.

The following is a chest specialization program that you can perform to develop size and symmetry in the pectoral muscles. Exercise substitutions can be made after Week #1, but perform the exercises according to the prescribed sets and reps. Follow this program for 2-3 weeks.

Chest Specialization Program

Workout #1

Chest Compound Set:
1) 20° DB press (6-8 reps)
2) Pushups (as many reps as possible)
- Perform 3 compound sets
- Rest 3 minutes between compound sets

Machine Flyes (3 sets of 10-12 reps, 2 minutes rest)

Workout #2

Guillotine press (3 sets, 10-12 reps, 90 seconds rest)

Perform 3 sets of 6-8 reps with 90 seconds rest on the following:

- Quadriceps
- Hamstrings
- Calves
- Back
- Deltoids
- Biceps

Workout #3

Gironda dips:
- 10 sets of as many reps as possible
- Do not train to muscular failure
- Rest for 3 minutes between sets

Workout #4

Perform 3 sets of 6-8 reps with 90 seconds rest on the following:

- Quadriceps
- Hamstrings
- Calves
- Back
- Deltoids
- Biceps
- Abs

You can perform the sequence of workouts throughout the week in the following manner:

Option #1

Day 1 – Workout #1
Day 2 – off
Day 3 – Workout #2
Day 4 – off
Day 5 – Workout #3
Day 6 – Workout #4
Day 7 – off

Option #2

Day 1 – Workout #1
Day 2 – Workout #2
Day 3 – off
Day 4 – Workout #3
Day 5 – Workout #4
Day 6 – off
Day 7 – off

11

Branding a Pair of Horseshoes

XI. Branding a Pair of Horseshoes

The triceps are a muscle that's misunderstood by many bodybuilders. For example, in every gym there are beginners who just do pressdowns. Then there's the guy who wants some mass in his triceps, so he performs nothing but close grip bench presses and dips. Then there's the guy who performs lying triceps extensions to the forehead with the wrong tempo.

Listen, nobody ever got big triceps off of pressdowns alone. You're a fool to believe that close grip presses and dips are the keys to massive triceps. And any idiot who performs skull crushers with quick, brisk reps should add a 100 more pounds on that EZ-curl bar and let it crush his puny little brain of his!

Wheww! Sorry. As you can tell, I'm in the middle of my dieting phase. Seriously though, most bodybuilders don't know how to develop massive triceps to balance out their biceps. Even Arnold had to play catch-up with his triceps to balance out his incredibly peaked bi's.

"So, Mr. Know It All, what's the big secret to massive triceps?"

First, I don't know it all; nobody does. Anyone who says he does is trying to sell you something. Second, it's not a big secret, but a bunch of little secrets that make up triceps size. If you want to discover these secrets, however, you should understand the differences between the different triceps heads.

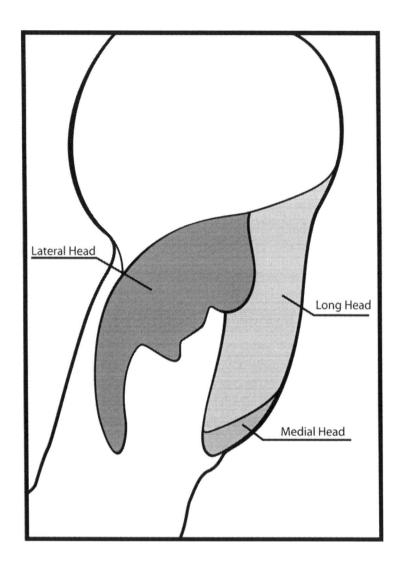

The Triceps Long Head

The triceps consists of three head: long, lateral and medial. The lateral head is on the outside of your upper arm just above your elbow. The triceps medial head is in between the lateral and long head. The long head is on the inside of your upper arm.

Do a biceps pose and look in the mirror. If the long head of your triceps is well developed, then the bottom of your upper arm should be curving downward, provided that you're not fat.

Most bodybuilders don't know how to properly develop the long head of their triceps, which is the meatiest portion. The lateral and medial heads are easily accessed whenever you perform any pressing movements, whether its bench presses, pressdowns, military presses, pushups or dips.

The long head, however, is not activated very much by presses. I don't care what MRI or EMG studies say. None of the aforementioned exercises activate the long head, not even dips, which is a supposed mass builder.

This is why when you select triceps exercises you should perform at least two: an extension movement for the long head and a pressing movement for the lateral and medial heads. Anyone who performs solely close grip presses or dips in the hopes of attaining thick, full triceps will be sorely disappointed.

To access the triceps long head, you must do the following:

1. Choose the appropriate exercise
2. Complete the appropriate number of reps
3. Execute the appropriate tempo
4. Take the appropriate amount of rest in between sets

1. Choosing Exercises

Of the three triceps heads (lateral, medial, and long head), the long head of the triceps is the meatiest of the three. Even when the lateral and medial heads are fully developed and the long head is underdeveloped, the long head is still comparable in size.

Whereas the lateral and medial heads have a mix of fast and slow-twitch fibers, the long head is comprised primarily of fast-twitch fibers. So when the fibers of the triceps long head are properly stressed, they develop tremendous size.

Exercises targeting the long head are 1) lying flat bench triceps extensions with an EZ curl bar and 2) lying decline extensions with an EZ curl bar. If you perform either one of these extension movements in conjunction with a pressing movement, then you will develop thick, full triceps.

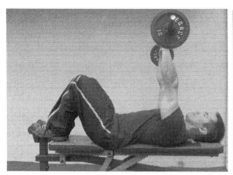 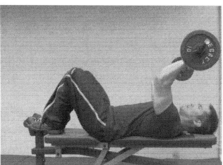

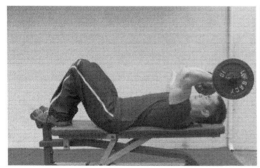 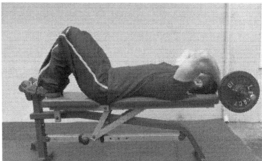

Lying Triceps Extensions (flat bench)

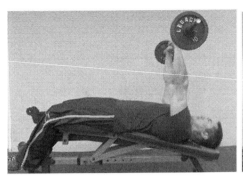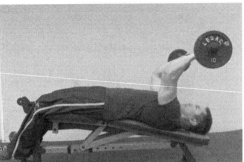
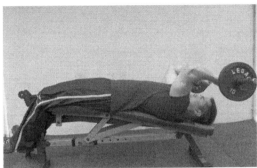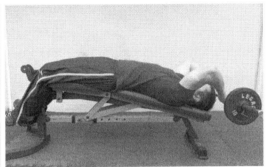

Lying Triceps Extensions (decline bench)

Keep in mind that you should perform lying extensions with an EZ-curl bar to keep the emphasis on the triceps long head. Performing lying triceps extensions with a straight barbell or dumbbells, however, will shift the emphasis to the lateral heads.

2. Rep Range

The long head of the triceps responds only to high loads, because it's composed mostly of fast-twitch muscle fibers. Whereas the lateral and medial heads respond to a wide variety of reps, low to moderate reps for the long head would be appropriate. You'll have to experiment to find the appropriate rep protocols for you, but I find that a continuum of 4-8 reps with a 4-6 target rep range right for most bodybuilders.

3. Rest Periods

Because of its high fast-twitch makeup, working the long head requires longer rest periods. High threshold muscles like the triceps long require heavy weight and lower reps. Heavy weight requires longer rest between sets to allow for nervous system recovery. Three to four minutes between sets should be enough for the triceps long head.

4. Tempo

Almost all exercises for the long head require that you slow it down in order to feel any sort of tension from the movement. Always slow down the eccentric portion of the movement when performing lying triceps extensions.

You can always vary the speed of the eccentric. Just make sure the speeds are slow enough that you can feel the weight. As for the concentric portion of these movements, you can also vary the speed. Unlike the eccentric portion, however, you should perform the concentric portion at high speeds if you're using heavy weight. To reiterate:

- Eccentric: somewhat slow to super slow
- Concentric: moderate to explosive

The Triceps Lateral and Medial Head

While the long head contributes significantly to triceps size, developing the lateral head contributes to the muscle's toned look. When you wear a short sleeve T-shirt, it's the thickness of the triceps lateral head that people see and will be most impressed by.

Unlike the triceps long head (which is purely fast-twitch), the lateral and medial heads have a mixed fiber makeup. This means that they respond to a wide variety of reps. Everything from heavy super low reps (4-8) to super high reps (20-25+).

The following are exercises that develop the lateral and medial head of the triceps. I have indicated which exercises should be performed with high reps and which should be performed with low reps.

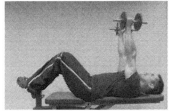 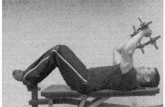 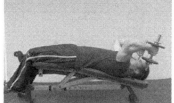

Lying dumbbell extensions – Lying triceps extensions with an EZ-curl bar primarily stress the triceps long head. Triceps extensions with dumbbells, however, stress all three triceps heads. This exercise can be performed with two dumbbells at the same time or one arm at a time.

Since lying dumbbell extensions work the long head as well as the lateral and medial heads, it's best to perform the exercise with a moderately heavy weight (4-8 reps). Use slow negatives, get a good stretch at the bottom and flex hard at the top.

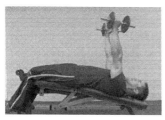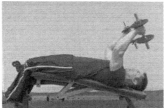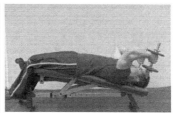

Decline dumbbell extensions — Like the flat bench version mentioned above, decline dumbbell extensions stress all three triceps heads. Just like the flat bench version, you should perform decline dumbbell extensions with moderately heavy weight (4-8 reps). Use slow negatives, get a good stretch at the bottom and flex hard at the top.

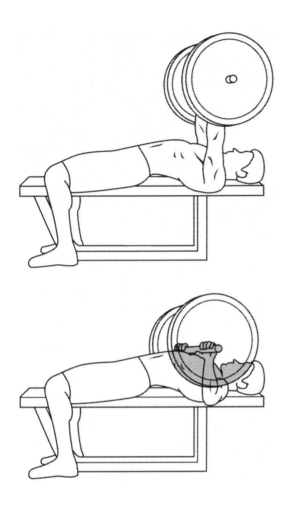

Close Grip Bench Press – Close grip bench presses will thicken the triceps lateral head. Load up enough weight to perform anywhere from 4-8 reps. Take a shoulder width and keep the elbows close to your torso. Be sure to lower the bar under control until it touches just above the nipple line. As you press up, be sure to push off explosively in a straight line every time.

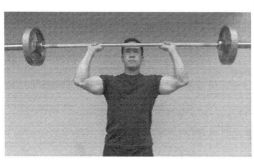 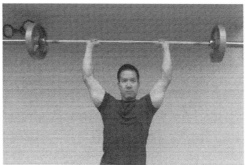

Standing overhead press (heavy partials) – All heavy partial presses develop thick triceps, but the standing overhead press will isolate the lateral and medial heads even more. Take a shoulder width grip on a barbell, position the bar at the top of your head and press it up until the bar is locked out directly above your head. Lower the bar slowly under control until it touches the top of head, then press it back up to lockout.

Essentially you use the top of your head as a reference point the same way you reference pins in a power rack. This will teach you to lower the bar under control and not bang your head with a weight that is too heavy. As you're pressing, keep your eyes straight ahead and your torso vertical. Tighten your abs and avoid overarching your lower back. Use a 4-8 rep max weight with this exercise.

Diamond pushups (feet elevated) - Place your hands on the floor and form a diamond shape. Raise your feet up on to a bench and perform as many pushups as you can. Use a brisk tempo: fast positive, fast negative.

If you can perform at least 13-15 reps, then this exercise is ideal for active recovery or back off sets. If you cannot perform a lot of reps on this exercise, then you can make it easier by performing it with the feet on the floor.

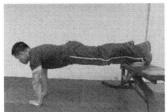 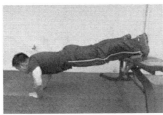 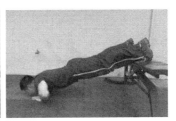

One-arm pushups – Although it is a difficult exercise to perform initially, the one-arm pushup will hit the lateral head very hard. Obviously you should be able to do a high number of regular two-handed pushups (40+) in good form before tackling the one-arm pushup.

If you've never performed one-arm pushups, then you may be discouraged by its difficulty. So what you have to do is perform and practice the intermediate exercises to one-arm pushups.

A good intermediary exercise is the "staggered pushup." This is where you perform pushups with one hand directly underneath your body and the other hand out to the side. Performing pushups in this manner places more emphasis on the arm directly underneath.

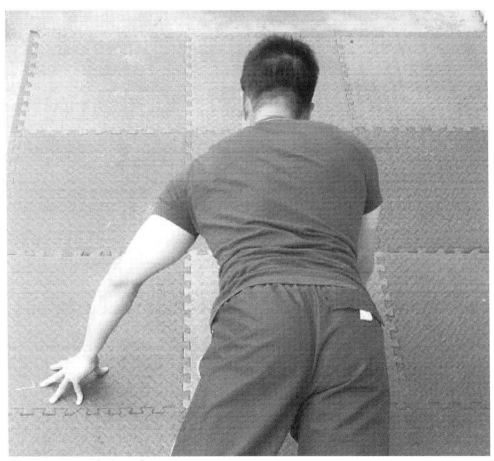

Staggered Pushup

Once you can perform a significant number of staggered pushups (10+), attempt the one-arm pushup. Widen your foot stance and place your pushup hand directly underneath your body. Place your free hand on the back of your leg. Tighten up your entire body, particularly your abs, lats and quads. Lower yourself under control and push up once you reach the floor.

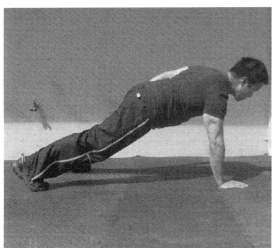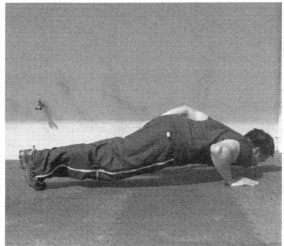

One Arm Pushup

Once you can do the wide stance one-arm pushup with relative ease, then you make it more difficult by placing your free hand behind your back and taking a narrow foot stance.

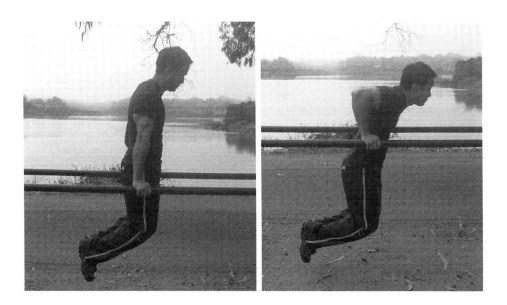

Dips – Parallel bar dips stress both the chest and triceps. If you have very strong triceps and can perform 15+ full range dips without difficulty, then dips will be a great active recovery exercise or an exercise to use as a back-off set.

If you find dips to be difficult, however, then simply perform them during the heavy low rep phases of your program. Do not perform bench dips, even though they're easier to perform. Bench dips tend to aggravate shoulder problems.

Compound Sets for the Triceps

Since the triceps is a horseshoe shaped muscle, bifurcated compound sets work well in bringing out triceps mass. The following is a triceps compound set that emphasizes the triceps long head:

1) Lying EZ-curl bar extensions (4-6 reps, fast positive/contract/slow negative) followed immediately by
2) Lying Dumbbell Extensions (6-8 reps, fast positive/contract/slow negative)

Perform 4 of these compound sets with 3-4 minutes rest. This compound set can also be done with the decline bench:

1) Decline EZ-curl bar extensions (4-6 reps, fast positive/contract/slow negative) followed immediately by
2) Decline Dumbbell Extensions (6-8 reps, fast positive/contract/slow negative)

Key Points on Triceps Training:

- Pressing movements work the lateral and medial triceps. Extension movements work the triceps long head.
- The triceps long head forms the bulk of triceps mass and size.
- The triceps long head is primarily fast-twitch and responds only to heavy weight, low reps and high rest.
- Thickening the triceps lateral head will give you muscle tone in the upper arm.

One last note on triceps training: always perform isotension on triceps. In other words, flex them in between sets and when you're not working out. This will help you exercise better muscle control, which translates to greater fiber recruitment when you hit the weights.

The following is a triceps specialization program that you can perform to develop thick triceps. Exercise substitutions can be made after Week #1, but perform the exercises according to the prescribed sets and reps. Follow this program for 2-3 weeks, and you'll have a pair of those lucky horseshoes in no time.

Triceps Specialization Program

Workout #1	Workout #2

Triceps Compound Set:
  1) Lying EZ-curl bar extensions (4-6 reps) followed immediately by
  2) Lying Dumbbell Extensions (6-8 reps)
  • Perform 4 compound sets
  • Rest 3-4 minutes between compound sets
	Arms Triset:
	  1) Lying dumbbell curls (6-8 reps)
	  2) Seated dumbbell curls (as many reps as possible with the same weight used for lying dumbbell curls)
	  3) Diamond pushups (as many reps as possible)
	  • Perform 3 trisets
	  • Rest 1 minute between trisets
	
	Perform 3 sets of 6-8 reps with 90 seconds rest for the following:
	
	  • Quads
	  • Hamstrings
	  • Back
	  • Chest
	  • Delts
	  • Calves

Workout #3	Workout #4

Close grip bench press:
  • 10 sets of 4-6 reps
  • Rest for 3 minutes between sets
	Perform 3 sets of 6-8 reps with 90 seconds rest for the following:
	
	  • Quads
	  • Hamstrings
	  • Back
	  • Chest
	  • Delts
	  • Biceps
	  • Calves

You can perform the sequence of workouts throughout the week in the following manner:

Option #1

Day 1 – Workout #1
Day 2 – off
Day 3 – Workout #2
Day 4 – off
Day 5 – Workout #3
Day 6 – Workout #4
Day 7 – off

Option #2

Day 1 – Workout #1
Day 2 – Workout #2
Day 3 – off
Day 4 – Workout #3
Day 5 – Workout #4
Day 6 – off
Day 7 – off

Biceps:
The Pinnacle of Brawn

XII. Biceps: The Pinnacle of Brawn

Quick! Make a muscle!

What did you do? You flexed your biceps, of course. The bicep is the symbol of strength and brawn. Biceps training is fun to do, because you get a sense of immediate gratification. There is something very satisfying about feeling and watching your arms bulge as you pump them up.

Angles, angles, angles!

The biceps is very sensitive to different angles of movement. Because of joint angles, the force or difficulty of a bicep curl varies along its range of motion. As mentioned in previous chapters, this is known as a "force curve" or "strength curve."

For example, performing incline curls will give you quite a different feel in the biceps as opposed to concentration curls. Incline curls will be harder at the bottom range of motion, while concentration curls will be more difficult at the top range of motion.

Because of this angle sensitivity, the biceps love a variety of exercises. For maximum development, you'll need to concern yourself with three angles to attack the biceps force curve:

1) Bottom range emphasis
2) Midrange emphasis
3) Top range emphasis

Bottom Range Exercises

Incline curls - Lie on an incline bench with dumbbells in both of your hands and your arms hanging down. Keeping your palms up and your elbows steady, curl the dumbbells up toward your deltoids. Control the movement and do not allow your elbows to move up. Then lower the dumbbells back toward the floor and get a good stretch on you biceps at the bottom.

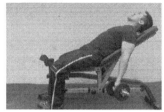 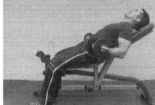 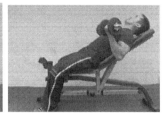

Lying dumbbell curls - To perform lying dumbbell curls lie on your back on a flat bench with dumbbells in both of your hands. Allow your arms to hang down but do not let the dumbbells make contact with the floor. As you keep your palms up and your elbows steady, curl the dumbbells up toward your deltoids. Control the movement at all times and do not allow your elbows to move up. Then lower the dumbbells back toward the floor and get a good stretch on you biceps at the bottom.

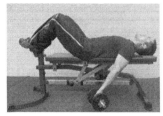 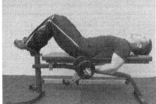 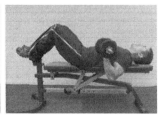

Lying dumbbell curls give you a great bicep stretch and provide constant tension in the muscles throughout the entire range of motion. Due to the angle of movement, the biceps must contract completely to compensate for the pull of gravity.

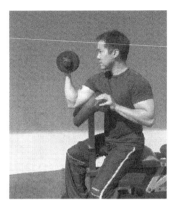 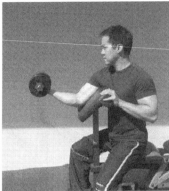 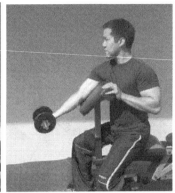

Preacher curls – This exercise will hit the brachialis. Sit at a preacher bench, place your arms on the angled padding and curl a weight up. You can use dumbbells or a barbell. You can perform them one-handed or two-handed. What's most important is that you straighten your arms fully as you lower the weight.

Midrange Exercises

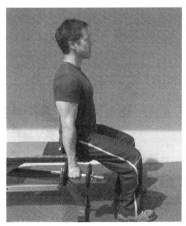 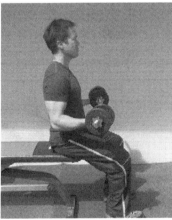 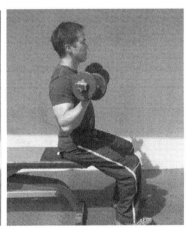

Seated dumbbell curls – Grab a pair of dumbbells and sit at the end of a bench, maintaining an upright position. Curl the weight up with an underhand grip.

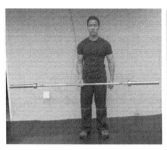 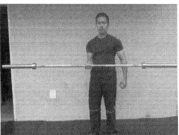 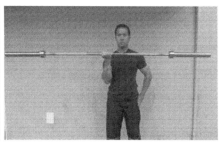

One Arm Barbell Curls - To perform this exercise, grab a barbell with one hand and perform one arm barbell curls. Make sure the barbell is parallel with the floor at all times. Doing barbell curls in this manner forces you to concentrate much harder on your grip and your biceps because of the greater balance and coordination involved.

Top Range Exercises

Exercises which stress the top range also develop biceps peak. Top range exercises work the brachialis, a golf ball sized muscle underneath your biceps near the inside of your elbow.

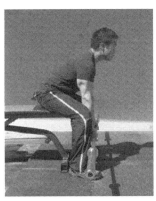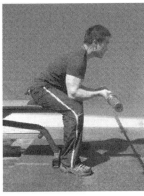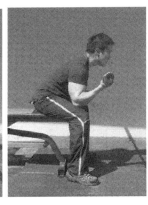

Barbell concentration curls – Sit at the end of a bench and lean forward, placing your elbows on top of your knees. Maintaining this position, grab a barbell and curl the weight up.

Barbell curls with chains – Since the force curve varies along a barbell curl, a great way to even out this force curve is to add chains to a barbell. As you curl, more and more links come off the floor. The weight becomes heavier and heavier as you lift. This is a form of "accommodating resistance," and it is an excellent way of increasing your strength. If you train with chains for a few weeks, and then train without them for the next few weeks, then your pounds will go up significantly.

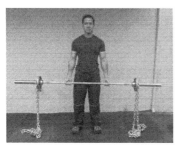 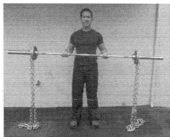 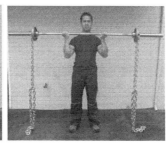

You can purchase chains at a hardware store, but very few have the really big ones needed for powerlifting. I got mine at Osh Orchard Supply and Hardware. If you want to add chains to your exercises, then you'll need the following:

- A pair of 3/8" chains, 5 feet long each (these are the lead chains; you'll loop these on to the barbell)
- A pair of 5/8" chains, 5 feet long each (you'll loop and hang these off the lead chains)
- Four carabiners to loop and attach the chains

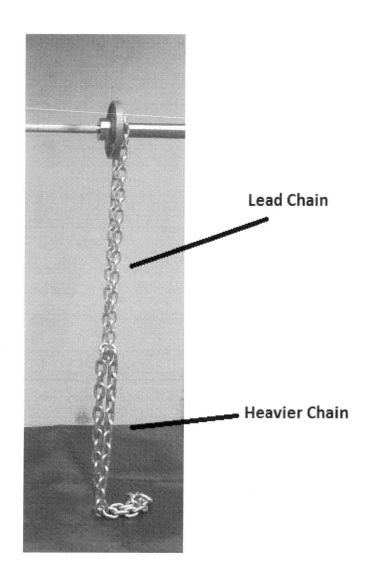

Lead Chain

Heavier Chain

You can also add chains to other barbell exercises such as squats, bench presses and seated military presses. Powerlifters use chains to break plateaus in strength development. If you train with chains for a few weeks, and then train without them for the next few weeks, your weights will go up significantly.

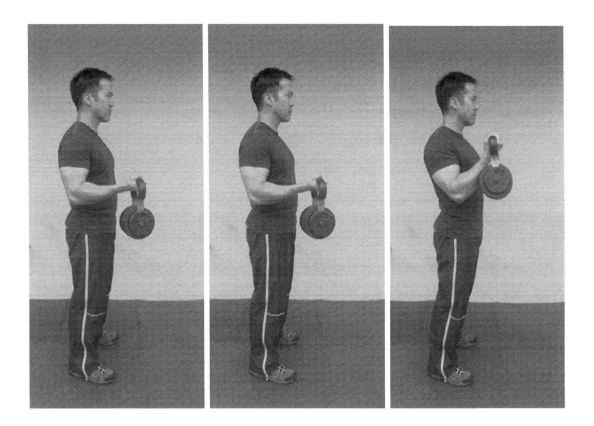

Kettlebell curls – Grab a kettlebell or two of moderate weight and curl them as you would curl a barbell or dumbbell. Since the kettlebell's center of gravity is outside of your palm, you will feel tension throughout the entire range of motion. Performed properly, this exercise will force peak contraction of the biceps.

Full Range Exercises

Certain biceps curls defy category. Exercises such as the "perfect curl" and the body drag curl involve moving your elbows and torso and will hit the biceps at 2 or more angles.

Perfect curls – This exercise requires you to shift your body around *while* you are lifting the weight. This is done to maintain a high level of muscular tension on the biceps throughout the entire range of motion.

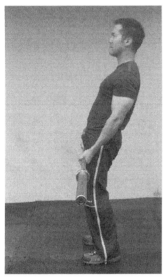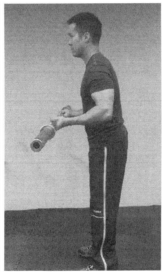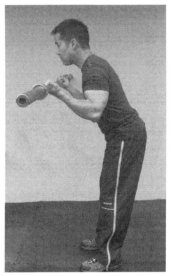

Stand holding a barbell with an underhand grip. Bend at the knees and lean back, keeping your torso in line with your upper thighs. From this position curl the weight up.

As you curl the weight up, slowly bend the upper torso forward so that your shoulders and elbows are in front of you. Contract hard at the top. Slowly lower the bar and reverse the entire sequence of movements.

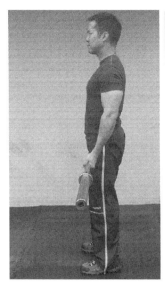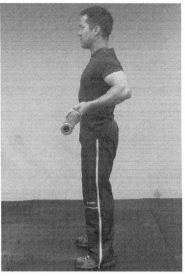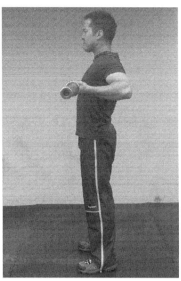

Body drag curls – Standing hold a barbell. Lift the weight straight up not by curling but by dragging the bar up along your body and raising your elbows back. The bar must be kept in contact with the body at all times. Squeeze hard at the top to get peak contraction. You can use either an underhand or overhand grip.

Target the Brachialis to Develop Biceps Peak

The brachialis is a golf ball sized muscle situated underneath your biceps next to the inside of your elbow. With regards to symmetry, this is a strategic pivot point on your arm. Develop the brachialis, and its increased size will push the biceps up and give you greater biceps "peak." Greater biceps peak adds to greater arm girth.

While your biceps have a mix of fast and slow-twitch fibers, the misnamed "lower biceps" or brachialis is composed primarily of fast-twitch fibers. Hence the brachialis responds best to heavy weight and low reps with fast positives and slow negatives.

The brachialis is activated when:

1) You perform curls with the elbows in the front of your body.
2) You perform curls with a neutral (hammer fist) grip or with a pronated (overhand) grip.

The following are exercises which develop the brachialis muscle:

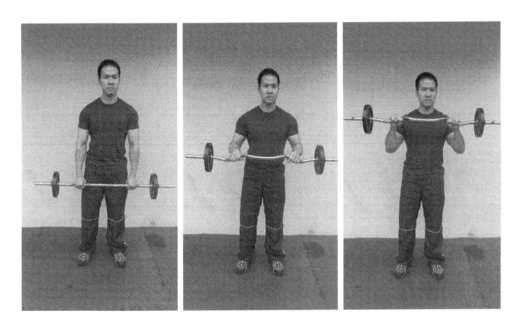

Reverse grip barbell curl – Stand holding an EZ-curl bar with an overhand grip. Curl the weight up explosively. Lower the weight slowly under control.

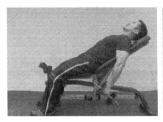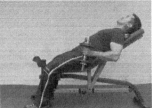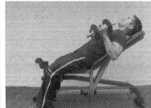

Incline hammer curls - Lie on an incline bench with your arms hanging down and holding a pair of dumbbells. Curl the dumbbells up toward your deltoids with a hammer fist grip. Control the movement and do not allow your elbows to move up. Then lower the dumbbells back toward the floor and get a good stretch on you biceps at the bottom.

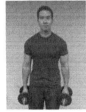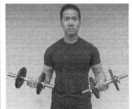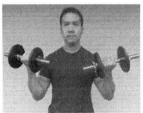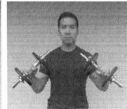

Zottman curls - To perform Zottman curls, simply take a pair of dumbbells in either a standing or seated position and curl them up. Once you've curled them to the top position, rotate your wrists so that your hands are pronated and your palms are facing the floor. From this position, lower the dumbbells slowly. Once you reach the bottom, repeat this method of curling and lowering for the desired number of reps. The Zottman curl is an excellent movement that works the brachialis, bicep, and forearm.

Priming the Pump: Trisets for Biceps

Hitting the biceps at different angles allows you to stress different portions of the force curve. A great way to incorporate the different angles and emphasize the entire force curve is to perform trisets for the biceps. Simply choose three biceps exercises (one emphasizing each range of the force curve) and perform them in sequence.

The following are some of my favorite triset combinations to pump up the biceps:

1. Incline dumbbell curls (bottom range)
2. Seated dumbbell curls (midrange)
3. Barbell concentration curls (top range)

1. Lying dumbbell curls (bottom range)
2. Seated dumbbell curls (midrange)
3. Barbell concentration curls (top range)

1. Zottman curls (midrange and brachialis)
2. Lying dumbbell curls (bottom range)
3. Perfect curls (full range)

1. Incline hammer curls (bottom range and brachialis)
2. Seated dumbbell curls (midrange)
3. Body drag curls (full range)

Mix it up!

To get big biceps, you must attack them from a variety of angles and grips. So head out to gym and mix it up! The key points on biceps training:

- The biceps are sensitive to variations on angle and grip.
- Attack the entire strength curve to grow the biceps: bottom, midrange, top.
- Hit the brachialis to develop biceps peak. The brachialis is comprised of purely fast-twitch fibers, so use heavy weight and low reps with a fast positive and slow negative.
- Underhand curling hits the biceps. Overhand and neutral grip curling hits the brachialis.

The following is a biceps specialization program that you can perform to build bigger biceps. Exercise substitutions can be made after Week #1, but perform the exercises according to the prescribed sets and reps. Follow this program for 2-3 weeks.

Biceps Specialization Program

Workout #1	Workout #2
Biceps Triset: 1) Incline hammer curls (6-8 reps) 2) Seated dumbbell curls (6-8 reps) 3) Barbell concentration curls (4-6 reps) • Perform 3 trisets • Rest 3 minutes between trisets	Arms Triset: 1. Lying dumbbell curls (6-8 reps) 2. Seated dumbbell curls (as many reps as possible with the same weight used for lying dumbbell curls) 3. Diamond pushups (as many reps as possible) • Perform 3 trisets • Rest 1 minute between trisets Perform 3 sets of 6-8 reps with 90 seconds rest for the following: • Quads • Hamstrings • Back • Chest • Delts • Calves
Workout #3 Zottman curls: • 10 sets of 4-6 reps • Fast positive, slow negative • Rest 3 minutes between sets	**Workout #4** Perform 3 sets of 6-8 reps with 90 seconds rest for the following: • Quads • Hamstrings • Back • Chest • Delts • Biceps • Calves

You can perform the sequence of workouts throughout the week in the following manner:

Option #1

Day 1 – Workout #1
Day 2 – off
Day 3 – Workout #2
Day 4 – off
Day 5 – Workout #3
Day 6 – Workout #4
Day 7 – off

Option #2

Day 1 – Workout #1
Day 2 – Workout #2
Day 3 – off
Day 4 – Workout #3
Day 5 – Workout #4
Day 6 – off
Day 7 – off

13 Cattle Call

XIII. Cattle Call

Calves: there is no other body part in which genetics plays such an enormous role. Bodybuilders throughout the years have experimented with numerous methods to induce growth in the calves, from jump-roping to wearing crazy shoes to ultra-high reps. Not one, however, has come up with a routine or technique that consistently produces results for the average person. Until now...

O.K., maybe I'm being a little overly dramatic, but quite frankly, the techniques that I'm going to reveal to you are the best methods that I've developed for inducing growth in the calves. I have never come across techniques that even come close to these. If you employ these techniques intermittently (every other workout, at most), then you will see some definite improvements in your calf size.

I must emphasize this, however: you can use these methods only if you're an advanced bodybuilder who's been religiously training his or her calves for a few years. If you've never trained your calves before or have not pushed yourself to the limit in calf training, then explore various other calf training methods before employing these techniques

Descending Sets

The calves have a high amount of slow-twitch (Type I) muscle fiber and intermediate fast-twitch (Type IIa) muscle fibers. This is why runners have good calf development, despite all of their cardio-based training.

Due to this high proportion of Type I and IIa muscle fibers, descending sets work quite well for calf development. For example a trainee can perform descending sets on a standing calf machine.

If you exercise at home, however, then you may not have access to a calf machine. A very good substitute for the standing calf machine exercise is an exercise known as the "dumbbell calf raise."

I can't remember from whom I picked this exercise up from first: Dan Duchaine or Steve Holman. Regardless of who invented it or who discovered it, the dumbbell calf raise is the best calf exercise, bar none. Yes, they're even better than donkey calf raises.

You will need a series of dumbbells descending in weight, a calf block, and something stable to hold on to like an incline bench or a squat rack. Take a dumbbell in one hand and with the other hand, hold on to a heavy, stable piece of equipment. Place the foot from the same side as the weight onto the edge of a calf block.

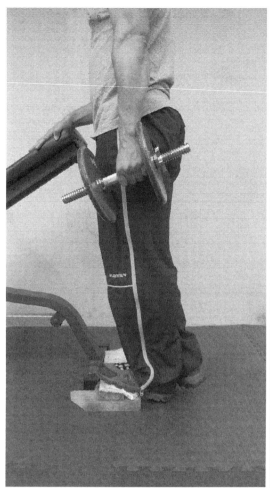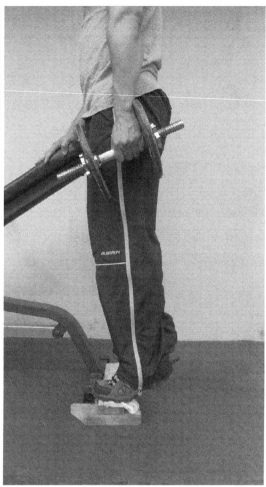

With that foot, and that foot alone, perform some calf raises. If your calf block is padded, then I suggest you perform the raises without any shoes. This will allow for greater range of motion, which means a deeper stretch and greater contraction for your calves.

To illustrate, if you're performing calf raises with your left foot first, then you would be holding the dumbbell at your side with your left hand. Your right hand would be holding on to something to maintain your balance. Your right foot wouldn't be touching anything at all.

There are two reasons why this exercise is so effective. First, the weight with which your calf is lifting (your body plus the dumbbell) is unstable.

Unless you're a ballerina, most people would find it difficult tiptoeing a dozen times on the edge of a block.

If you're new to the exercise, then performing it with your bodyweight alone will be difficult. The instability of the dumbbell calf raise makes it superior to the traditional standing machine calf raise, where the weight is stabilized.

The other reason for this exercise's effectiveness is that you're training one limb at a time, which is known as unilateral training. When one limb is forced to handle a weight by itself, your nervous system recruits more fibers in that muscle.

If you've never performed the dumbbell calf raise, then I suggest you train your calves with this exercise until you're no longer making any progress with it before moving on to the following set extension technique.

Descending Sets

O.K., now that you know how to perform the exercise, let's incorporate the shock technique known as "descending sets," otherwise known as "strip sets," "drop sets" or "down the rack." After you've warmed up your calves, grab a weight that will allow you to crank out 8-10 reps to failure on the dumbbell calf raise.

For example, work the right calf in a steady and continuous tempo, then switch the weight from your right hand to your left hand and immediately work the left calf with the same tempo. That's one strip set.

Once you're finished, immediately grab a lighter dumbbell and crank out another 8-10 reps to failure on your right calf, then on your left calf. That's a second strip set. Repeat this process two more times, for a total of four strip sets. On your fifth and final strip set, perform one-legged calf raises without a dumbbell. Rest for 2-3 minutes, and repeat the entire process with slightly less weight.

Here's how it would look step by step:

Dumbbell Calf Raises (For each set, alternate between your left and right calf without resting unless indicated)
1st set: 10-12 reps w/ 25 lb. Dumbbell
2nd set: 10-12 reps w/ 20 lb. Dumbbell
3rd set: 10-12 reps w/ 15 lb. Dumbbell
4th set: 10-12 reps w/ 10 lb. Dumbbell
5th set: 10-12 reps w/ bodyweight only
Rest 2 minutes
6th set: 10-12 reps w/ 20 lb. Dumbbell
7th set: 10-12 reps w/ 15 lb. Dumbbell
8th set: 10-12 reps w/ 10 lb. Dumbbell
9th set: 10-12 reps w/ 5 lb. Dumbbell
10th set: 10-12 reps w/ bodyweight only
> perform all sets to failure
> use a full range of motion
> use a steady and continuous tempo

In performing the above technique, you would have completed a total of 20 sets (10 for each calf) in only 5-8 minutes, assuming that you didn't rest at all between strip sets.

As you can see, it's a very intense technique. For this reason, I don't recommend employing this method all the time. Once a week is more than enough. For your other calf workouts, train them as you would normally train them.

Diminishing Sets

Most bodybuilders know of descending sets, but there is a lesser known technique that effectively hypertrophies slow-twitch dominant muscles. It's called "diminishing sets."

With diminishing sets, you choose a weight and strive to perform a total of 100 reps in the fewest number of sets possible. Typically, bodyweight-only exercises are chosen.

Diminishing sets can be performed on the calves by doing one-legged calf raises. With this exercise, you will perform bodyweight-only one-legged calf raises off the edge of a calf block. One hand will be holding on to a support of some sort. You will alternate between the left and right leg with little or no rest until you reach 100 reps on each calf. Start off a high number of reps at first, and then when your reps start falling below 10, rest for about 10 seconds and resume.

The burn that you get with this method is enough to make you limp for a week, but it's a brutally effective method to induce hypertrophy in the calves.

Key Points on Calf Training:

- The calf muscles are comprised primarily of slow-twitch and intermediate fast-twitch (Type IIa). They respond best to high reps (10+) with fast positives/fast negatives.
- Descending sets and diminishing sets can effectively build up the calves.

The following is a calf specialization program that you can perform for 2-3 weeks to develop the size of your calves. This program incorporates both descending sets (a.k.a. drop sets) and diminishing sets.

Do not perform this program unless you've been consistently training your calves for at least 6 months. Otherwise, your calves are going to be locked up in rigor mortis, and you'll be walking around on your tippy-toes. Don't even think about doing these workouts less than a week before an athletic event (unless you're a ballerina).

Calf Specialization Program

Workout #1

Calves Diminishing Sets:
- One legged calf raises (100 reps, bodyweight only, alternate between legs with no rest)

Quadriceps (3-4 sets of 6-8 reps, 90 seconds rest)

Hamstrings (3-4 sets of 6-8 reps, 90 seconds rest)

Workout #2

Perform 3-4 sets of 6-8 reps with 90 seconds rest for the following:

- Back
- Chest
- Deltoids
- Biceps
- Triceps
- Abs

Workout #3

Standing one legged calf raise (3 sets, as many reps as possible with body weight only, 60 seconds rest)

Perform 3 sets of 6-8 reps with 90 seconds rest for the following:

- Quadriceps
- Hamstrings
- Back
- Chest
- Deltoids
- Biceps
- Triceps

Workout #4

Dumbbell calf raises (2 series of 5 drop sets of 8-10 reps each, 2 minutes rest)

Perform 3 sets of 6-8 reps with 90 seconds rest for the following:

- Quadriceps
- Hamstrings
- Back
- Chest
- Deltoids
- Biceps
- Triceps

You can perform the sequence of workouts throughout the week in the following manner:

Option #1

Day 1 – Workout #1
Day 2 – Workout #2
Day 3 – off
Day 4 – Workout #3
Day 5 – off
Day 6 – Workout #4
Day 7 – off

Option #2

Day 1 – Workout #1
Day 2 – Workout #2
Day 3 – off
Day 4 – Workout #3
Day 5 – Workout #4
Day 6 – off
Day 7 – off

Carving out Boulder Shoulders

XIV. Carving out Boulder Shoulders

Everybody wants Steve Reeves' shoulders. His deltoid development wasn't exceptionally impressive, but he was blessed with a wide shoulder girdle that more than made up for any flatness in his deltoid muscles.

For us mere mortals, however, we have to work our shoulders to obtain some kind of width. I have narrow shoulders, so I've always paid special attention to developing my lateral delts.

To create the illusion of width in your shoulders, you should understand the differences between the three heads that comprise the deltoid muscle group.

The Anterior Head

This is the deltoid head you need to worry about the least. Most bodybuilders perform plenty of bench presses, incline presses, and military presses to develop this deltoid. Even when it comes to standing lateral raises, the anterior head will activate if you use poor form (which most people do).

Unless you're lacking in anterior head development, I would skip direct front deltoid training if you're solely a bodybuilder. Since they're mostly made up of fast-twitch fibers, heavy pressing (from any angle) will activate the anterior heads. If you already working the chest with presses, pushups and dips, then you're also working the front deltoids.

If you are lacking in anterior deltoid size, however, then do some overhead pressing. The following are pressing exercises that develop the front deltoids:

Standing Barbell Military Press - Stand and press the barbell up in line with your body. Many people press the weight up at a slight angle in front of their bodies. If you press the weight up and you can see your arms through your peripheral vision, then you've got poor alignment.

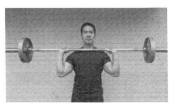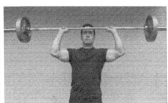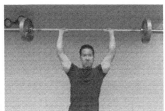

To remedy this, bring your arms back, squeeze your shoulder blades, and tighten your abs throughout the press. Your arms should be out of your peripheral vision as you lift. At the top of the press, the barbell should be directly over your head.

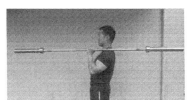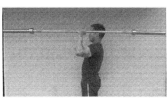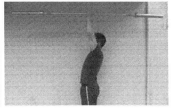

Javelin press – This is essentially a one-arm barbell press. Grab a barbell at the center with one hand and place it perpendicular to your shoulders. Press the barbell up without wobbling. The barbell should be aligned parallel to the floor at all times. This exercise will work your grip as well as thicken the triceps lateral head.

Kettlebell clean and press - Place a kettlebell between your feet. Bend down and grab the kettlebell with one hand. Explode up through the hips and raise the kettlebell to your shoulder. Press the kettlebell overhead.

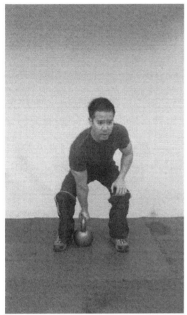 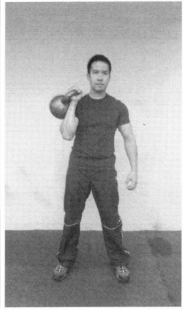 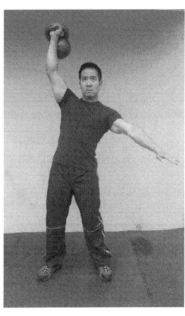

The kettlebell clean and press is not only a shoulder builder, but it is also an anabolic blowtorch. You will build a lot of overall muscle in the shoulders, back and arms if you use a heavy kettlebell. Five to seven reps is a good range to get the anabolic effect.

The Posterior Head

This is the least developed deltoid in bodybuilders. Although many bodybuilders perform bent-over lateral raises, this exercise is actually a poor choice for developing the posterior deltoid. With bent-over laterals, there is a tendency to cheat and swing the weights up with the help of the upper back muscles, the trapezius, and the legs.

The posterior deltoid is activated only in the top quarter range of the movement, and yet the amount of time spent in this crucial upper range is less than a second since most lifters swing the weights up. Bent-over laterals simply do not produce enough tension in the posterior deltoids.

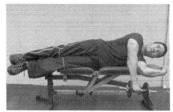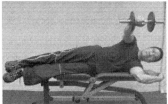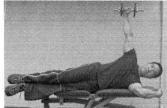

Side Lying Reverse Flyes – To develop the rear deltoids, I prefer the exercise known as "side lying reverse flyes." This is simply an exercise where you lie on your side and perform the rear delt raises one arm at a time. The lying reverse flye is a superior exercise, because it allows for a greater stretch of the posterior deltoid when the dumbbell passes across the chest and comes close to the floor.

The Lateral Head

This is the deltoid head that you want to focus on to create the illusion of width in shoulders. You want to develop the bulbous look of this head, so that you have some separation between it and your biceps and triceps. If your lateral head became flat, not only would you lose the illusion of wide shoulders, but your arms would also look fat if you had large biceps and triceps.

The lateral deltoids are comprised of primarily of Type I endurance fibers and Type II(a) intermediate fast-twitch fibers. In other words, the lateral fibers of the deltoid are meant for strength endurance. Hence the lateral deltoids grow on 3 factors:

    1) High reps (8+)
    2) Super low rest between sets (10 seconds to 1 minute)
    3) High frequency (at least 3 times per week)

You should complete a higher number of reps for the lateral head with little or no rest. The lateral deltoids grow very well on a set/rep pattern of 3-4 sets of 8-15 reps, 30-60 seconds rest periods, performed 3-4 times per week. Set extension techniques such trisets and descending sets work particularly well for the lateral head, since the lateral head is meant to handle a high volume of work.

The following exercises below will target the deltoid lateral head. Proper technique and form are essential to building the lateral deltoid. If your form is off in any way, then these exercises will instead work your front deltoids or your trapezius.

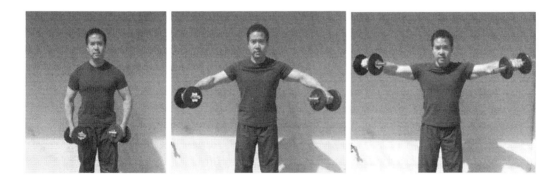

Standing lateral raises – Stand holding a pair of dumbbells in front of you. Raise the dumbbells up with the arms slightly bent. Do not raise the arms directly out to the sides, but to the sides and slightly out in front. In other words, raise your arms out to the 10 o'clock and 2 o'clock positions.

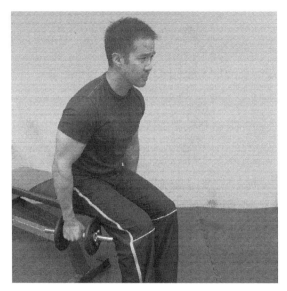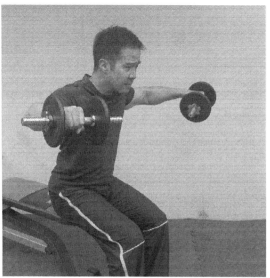

Seated lateral raises – Laterals can also be performed seated. Sit at the end of a bench with a slight lean forward and the dumbbells held under your thighs. With your arms slightly bent, raise the dumbbells out to the sides, but slightly in front of your body.

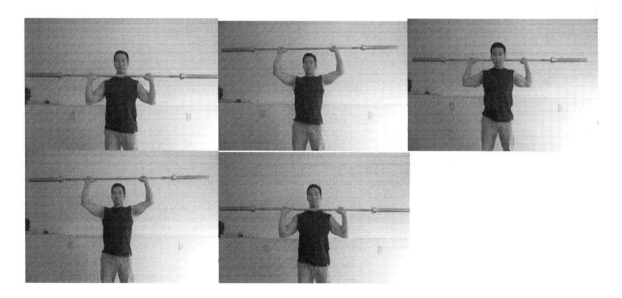

Bradford press – This is also known as a "Rocky press" or a "rainbow press." Hold the barbell in front of you with a wider than shoulder width grip and press up. Once the bar clears the top of your head, lower the bar behind your neck. Press the bar back up and once it clears the top of your head, lower it back to the front of your shoulders. This is one rep. Avoid locking out the arms, since this will shift the tension to the triceps. Keep alternating between pressing from the front and back until you reach the target repetitions.

This exercise places constant tension on your shoulders. Since Bradford presses work the lateral and anterior delts, you should perform a higher number of repetitions. A good target rep range would be 10-12 reps.

Dumbbell lateral swings- Vince Gironda developed some odd exercises, and this is one of the odder ones. But believe me, it works. Take a pair of dumbbells like you normally do for standing laterals. Raise both dumbbells up to shoulder level towards one side of your body, as if you were drawing a bow and arrow.

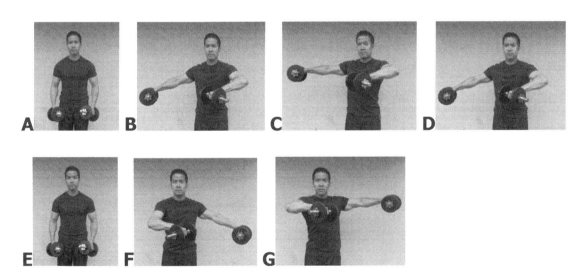

Bring the dumbbells down and raise them towards the opposite direction, again as if you were an archer drawing a bow. Keep your palms face down at the top of each swing. Like a pendulum, try to maintain a smooth and continuous motion from side to side as you switch positions.

Wide grip upright rows- Although this is not a lateral movement, it is essentially a barbell variation of standing dumbbell laterals. This exercise is not the same as conventional standing upright rows, where you take a narrow grip and pull it close to the body. Narrow grip upright rows stress the trapezius muscle and not the deltoids. Your goal as a bodybuilder is to develop thick, round delts but *minimize* trap development. Large traps will make your shoulders look narrow.

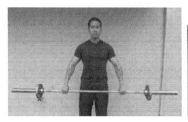 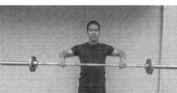 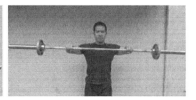

To perform wide grip upright rows, take a standing position and hold a barbell at mid-thigh. Make sure you have an overhand shoulder-width grip on the barbell. Pull the barbell up to a position about 10 inches in front of the middle of your chest. At this top position, your elbows should be on the same level as or higher than that of the barbell. If you've performed it correctly, the movement should resemble dumbbell lateral raises but with a barbell.

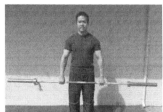 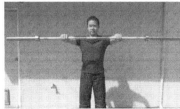 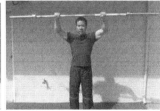

Barbell high pulls – This is Vince Gironda's version of the high pull, which is different from the version Olympic weightlifters perform. Stand holding a barbell with an overhand grip about shoulder-width apart. Pull the bar up until it is raised to about the top of your head. At this top position, the bar should be about 12 inches in front of the head.

Scott Press -- This exercise places continuous tension on all three deltoid heads. Grab a pair of dumbbells that you would normally use for laterals. Hold them in front of you, as if you're about to complete a biceps curl, with the elbows slightly forward.

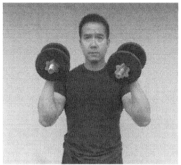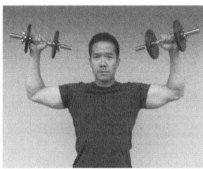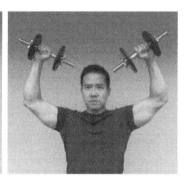

From this position, move your arms out to the sides till it looks like you're forming a "W." At this point, press the dumbbells up in an arc, keeping your elbows as far back as possible. That's one rep. Now slowly reverse the movement and perform 8-12 reps. Make sure you perform this entire movement slowly. This will give you a burn in your shoulders that you've never felt before.

You can perform the Scott press standing or seated at the end of a bench. Do not perform the Scott press sitting in a chair with back support, since you would lean back for support and this would shift the focus to your front delts.

The Rotator Cuff

Stability is the foundation of strength. Strength is the foundation of size. Therefore, if you want to have massive shoulders, then you'll need to ensure the stability of your shoulder joint.

To stabilize your shoulder joint, you'll need to do exercises which strengthen the rotator cuff. Rotator cuff work will not only stabilize your shoulders and increase your strength, but it will also improve your posture and widen the look of your shoulders by pulling them back into alignment.

People always use high reps for the rotator cuff, but the rotator cuff is comprised of tendons and fast-twitch muscle fiber. Hence, you'll get much better shoulder stabilization by using moderately heavy weight and moderate reps. What I recommend is to start off with light weight and pyramid your weights up until you're comfortably performing 6-8 reps.

The following are exercises that work the rotator cuff and stabilize your shoulders:

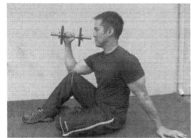 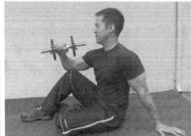 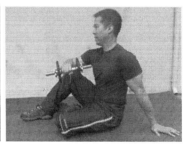

External Rotator on Knee - Sit with one knee propped up in front of you. With a dumbbell in hand, rest your elbow on top of your knee. Raise your arm and form an "L." From this position, slowly lower the dumbbell down under control, then raise it back up to the starting position.

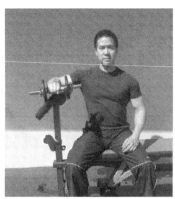 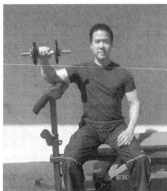 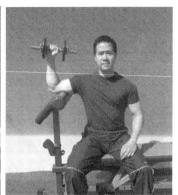

Propped External Rotator - Sit sideways on a preacher bench. With a dumbbell in hand, rest your elbow on the top of the preacher bench. Raise your arm and form an "L" out to the side. From this position, slowly lower the dumbbell down under control, then raise it back up to the starting position.

Kettlebell windmills - The kettlebell windmill will not only strengthen your rotator cuff, but it will also stretch hip flexors. Press a kettlebell overhead with one arm and lockout. Your feet should be pointed at a 45° degree angle away from the arm with the locked out kettlebell. While keeping your arm locked out overhead at all times, bend over to the opposite leg, pushing your hip out in the other direction.

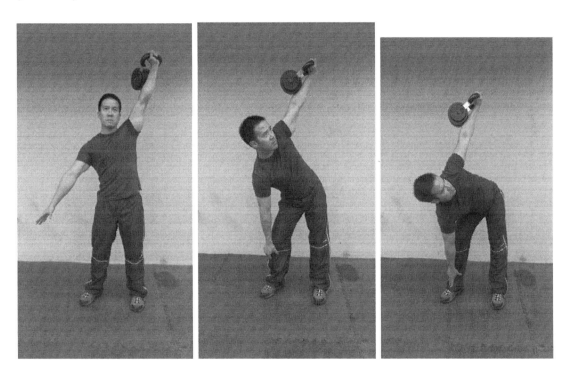

Lower yourself with the kettlebell locked out until your free hand touches the floor or your foot. Pause for one second and reverse the movement until you're back in the standing position.

Key Points on Deltoid Training

If you still can't get boulder shoulders after blasting away with these exercises, then you're out of luck. But hey, who knows? Maybe those shoulder pads from the 80's will be in fashion again.

Just remember:

- Target the lateral and posterior deltoids to emphasize shoulder width. The front deltoid gets enough work from presses for the chest.
- The lateral head is composed primarily of slow-twitch (Type I) and intermediate fast-twitch fibers (Type IIa). The lateral head responds best to high reps (8+), low rest periods (10-60 seconds) and high frequency of training (3-4 times per week).
- Strengthen your shoulders by strengthening the rotator cuff.

The following is a deltoid specialization program that you can perform to develop shoulder width. Exercise substitutions can be made after Week #1, but perform the exercises according to the prescribed sets and reps. Follow this program for 2-3 weeks.

Shoulders Specialization Program

Workout #1

Deltoid Compound Set:
1) Bradford press (10-12 reps)
2) Wide grip upright rows (perform as many reps as possible with the same weight used in the Bradford press)
- Perform 3 compound sets.
- Rest 2 minutes between compound sets.

Workout #2

Perform 3 sets of 6-8 reps with 90 seconds rest for the following:

- Quadriceps
- Hamstrings
- Calves
- Chest
- Back
- Biceps
- Triceps

Workout #3

Seated laterals (4 sets, 10-12 reps, 30 seconds rest)

Perform 3 sets of 6-8 reps with 90 seconds rest for the following:

- Quadriceps
- Hamstrings
- Calves
- Chest
- Back
- Biceps
- Triceps

Workout #4

Scott press (6 sets, 6-8 reps, 10-20 seconds rest)

Perform 3 sets of 6-8 reps with 90 seconds rest for the following:

- Quadriceps
- Hamstrings
- Calves
- Chest
- Back
- Biceps
- Triceps

You can perform the sequence of workouts throughout the week in the following manner:

Option #1

Day 1 – Workout #1
Day 2 – Workout #2
Day 3 – off
Day 4 – Workout #3
Day 5 – off
Day 6 – Workout #4
Day 7 – off

Option #2

Day 1 – Workout #1
Day 2 – Workout #2
Day 3 – off
Day 4 – Workout #3
Day 5 – Workout #4
Day 6 – off
Day 7 – off

Razor Sharp Abs

XVI. Razor Sharp Abs

Six-pack abs: everybody wants them. It doesn't matter if you're a man or woman, bodybuilder or MMA fighter, weekend warrior or a housewife with kids. Everybody wants abs they can shred cheese on. Everybody wants the six-pack, because abs symbolize both strength and sexual appeal.

Unfortunately, most people go about the wrong way training for six-pack abs. People think that if they did hundreds of crunches and sit-ups, that it will melt away the love handles. Of course the concept of spot reduction is a bunch of B.S., and yet people keep buying into this garbage.

Spot reduction on the abs is close to impossible, because the range of motion for most ab exercises is so short, that these exercises don't burn enough calories by themselves to make any impact on your physique. The amount of calories you burn with crunches is so low, that if you did 100 crunches a day and nothing else, you'd end up with a distended gut: toned six-pack underneath a layer of fat. You can't burn fat off your love handles with just ab work.

The second thing is that waistline fat is stubborn fat and is the last place to be burned off on men. When your body is in fat-burning mode, it will burn the fat from the limbs first, from the torso second, and (if you're a guy or a woman with a hormonal imbalance) from the waist LAST.

You have to diet, do cardio intervals, and do whole body strength training. That will burn off fat from your entire body and will eventually burn away your love handles. There is no such thing as spot reduction for the abs, because spot reduction for the abs is really just total body fat loss. In other words, you have to use whole body movements such as sprinting or clean and jerks to burn fat overall and burn fat from the stomach area.

What's more is that you're more likely to overtrain when you perform exercises that target the abs. The reason is that there is a large network of nerves in your core area. This is why people feel the wind knocked out of them when they get punched or kneed in the stomach and in the solar plexus.

Overstimulating this network of nerves in the abdominals will exhaust your nervous system and as a result, you're more likely to overtrain and compromise your efforts to gain muscular size. If you're an ectomorph training to gain muscle mass, then direct ab work is not necessary.

Rather than isolate your abs with direct work, you can work your abs by *integrating* your abs into compound exercises that you perform for other muscle groups. Simply tense your abs for multi-joint exercises such as pull-ups, front squats and military presses.

Tightening the abs and bringing them in to make your stomach flat while performing these exercises will stabilize your core. This is a form of isometrics that will develop myogenic tone, but not overdevelop the abs.

Your abs will develop a more "cut" look, if you diet and train correctly. This means low carb dieting and whole body movements with minimal rest (30-60 seconds). The abs will look like they're etched in, rather than popping out.

If you do a lot of direct work for the abs, like crunches or sit-ups, then your abs will overdevelop and protrude outward. You'll have rolls of abs instead of carved abs.

If you're an endomorph who's lost a considerable amount of weight from the waist, however, then you'll benefit more from direct ab work. Direct ab work will tighten the waistline stretched out from years of obesity.

Exercise Selection for the Abs

For complete development of any muscle, you only need 2 carefully selected exercises. The abdominal muscles are no different. To fully work the abs, you need an exercise that works the rectus abdominus (the six-pack) and one that works the transverse abdominus, which is hidden underneath the rectus abdominus.

Most people focus on the six-pack or the rectus abdominus and do endless crunches, flutter kicks and sit-ups. Yet when it comes to posture and shrinking your waistline, it's really the unseen transverse abdominus that is important.

The transverse abdominus lies underneath the six-pack and is responsible for bringing your stomach in, as well as stabilizing your torso. Thus, when you tighten the transverse abdominus, you instantly have a thinner waist and straightened posture.

Here are 5 exercises that strengthen the transverse abdominus, the six-pack or both:

1) **Planks** (transverse abdominus)

- Place your hands and feet on the floor as if you were going to perform a pushup. But instead of performing a pushup, simply hold that position for as long as you can.
- Keep your head, torso and legs straight and aligned with each other.
- Tighten your abs, triceps, and thighs, and do not let your stomach and hips sag. If they do, then that is the end of the set.

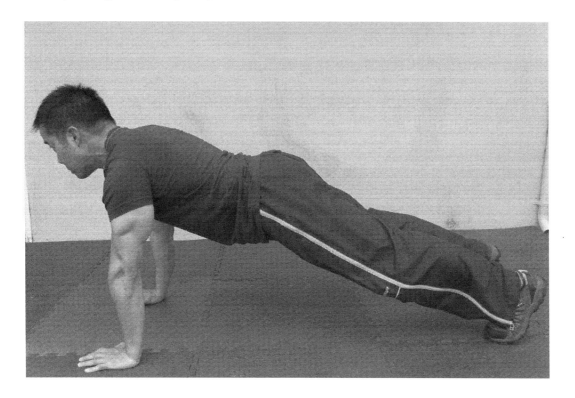

Most athletes, however, can easily perform the Plank. After all, this is simply the starting position for the pushup. With proper training and practice, most people will perform the Plank with very little difficulty. Once you achieve the Plank, progress to the harder version: one arm up and one leg up.

To perform this advanced version, get into Plank position. Raise one arm up. Then raise the opposite leg and keep both limbs up and aligned with your body. So if you raise your right hand, then you would simultaneously raise your left leg.

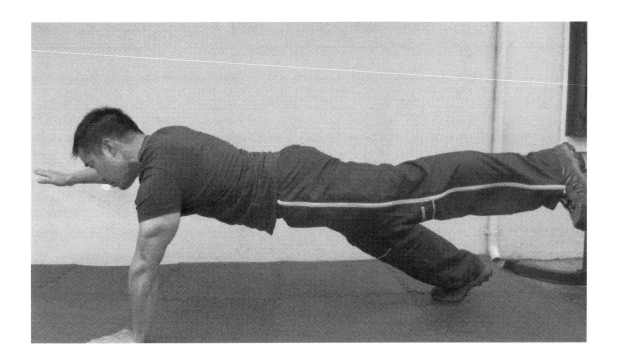

- Keep your raised arm and leg straight and aligned with your body. Maintain this position for as long as you can.
- Being in this precarious position requires even greater concentration than a normal Plank. Tighten your abs, triceps, and thighs, and do not drop your arm or leg from their raised positions. When you lose your balance, then that is the end of the set.
- Repeat for the opposite arm and leg.

2) Stomach Vacuum (transverse abdominus)

- To do the stomach vacuum, exhale all the air out of your lungs and bring your stomach in as far as it can go.
- Once your stomach is sucked as far as it can go, hold that position and continue to breathe shallow breaths through the mouth. Each time you exhale, bring your navel closer and closer to your spine.
- When you can no longer hold this position, release and breathe regularly for a few seconds.
- Repeat for three to five reps. Each isometric hold is considered one repetition.

3) The Front Lever (transverse abdominus)

- Grab a bar, raise your body until it's in a horizontal position and parallel with the floor.
- Keep your arms straight and simply hold this position for as long as you can.
- To maintain this static hold, you will need to tighten your entire body: abs, lats, glutes and quads.

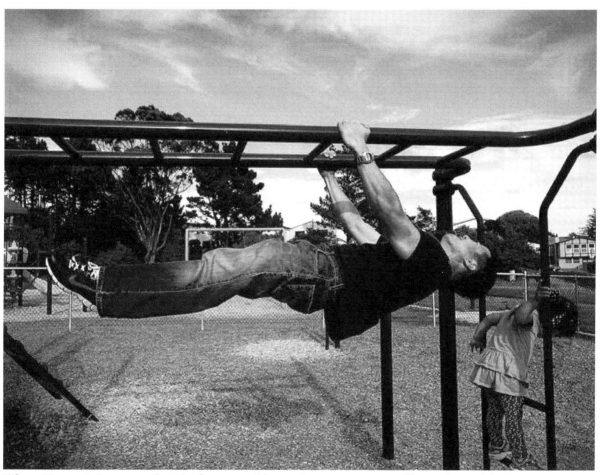

The Front Lever (with future Olympic gymnast off to the side)

4) Hanging Leg Raises (rectus abdominus and transverse abdominus)

- With an overhand shoulder width grip grab an overhead bar and hang.
- Tighten your grip and flex your lats and abs.
- Curl your trunk and slowly raise your feet up to the bar, keeping your legs semi-straight.
- Try not to lean back as you raise your legs to the bar. As you raise your legs, try to curl your body in and "crunch" your abs.
- Lower your legs and repeat, keeping excess momentum to a minimum.

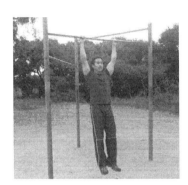 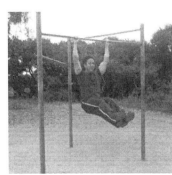 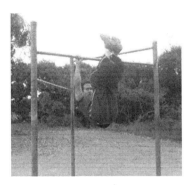

5) **Dragon Flags** (rectus abdominus and transverse abdominus)

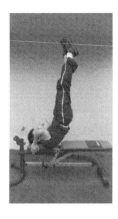 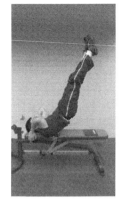 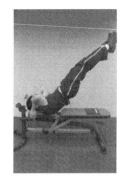 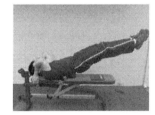

- Lie on a flat bench.
- Firmly grip the sides of the bench beneath your head.
- Keeping your head firmly on the bench, extend your legs straight out and raise them overhead pointing straight up to the ceiling. Keep your torso and legs straight and in line with each other as you raise them overhead.
- From this 90° position, slowly lower your legs and torso, keeping them in line the entire time.
- Repeat for as many repetitions as you can complete.

Key Points on Ab Training:

- There is no such thing as spot reduction. Doing ab exercises alone will not get you six-pack abs. To see your abs, you have to strip away body fat with low carb dieting and whole body movements with low rest periods.
- Classical bodybuilders desire abs that are etched in as opposed to popping out. To obtain this look, choose ab exercises where you isometrically contract your abs.

Since we want to avoid overdeveloping and over stimulating the abs, it's not necessary to designate an ab day or an ab specialization program. High volume will build up the abs and make them protrude outward. To minimize ab growth, we'll train them with low volume, high frequency.

To get ripped abs you have to be ripped throughout your entire body. The following is a fat loss program designed to get you lean and mean through strength training. A few sets of abs are done at every workout. Exercise substitutions can be made, but perform the exercises according to the prescribed sets and reps. Follow this program for 2-3 weeks.

Fat Loss Program

Workout #1	Workout #2
Barbell clean & press: • 5 sets of 5 reps • 90 second rest periods • Speed is more important than weight. Choose a moderately heavy weight and perform explosive reps in good form. **Superset:** 1) Pull-ups (as many reps as possible) 2) Back squats (10-12 reps) • Perform 3 supersets • Rest 90 seconds between supersets Hanging leg raises (3 sets, as many reps as possible, 90 seconds rest)	Planks (3 sets, 90 seconds rest) Deltoids (8 sets, 8 reps, 45 seconds rest) Biceps (8 sets, 8 reps, 45 seconds rest) Triceps (8 sets, 8 reps, 45 seconds rest) Calves (8 sets, 8 reps, 45 seconds rest)
Workout #3	Workout #4
Barbell clean & press: • 8 sets of 3 reps • 1 minute rest periods • Speed is more important than weight. Choose a moderately heavy weight and perform explosive reps in good form. **Superset:** 1) Deadlifts (4-6 reps) 2) Pushups (as many reps as possible) • Perform 5 supersets • Rest 90 seconds between supersets Hanging leg raises (3 sets, as many reps as possible, 90 seconds rest)	Planks (3 sets, 90 seconds rest) Deltoids (8 sets, 8 reps, 30 seconds rest) Biceps (8 sets, 8 reps, 30 seconds rest) Triceps (8 sets, 8 reps, 30 seconds rest) Calves (8 sets, 8 reps, 30 seconds rest)

Perform the sequence of workouts throughout the week in the following manner:

Day 1 – Workout #1
Day 2 – Workout #2
Day 3 – off
Day 4 – Workout #3
Day 5 – Workout #4
Day 6 – off
Day 7 – off

Follow a low carb diet while on this specialization program. This means no "white" or "brown" carbs of any sort. No pastas, breads, rice, sugar, dairy or alcohol. During this program, you should be eating "green" carbs, which are vegetables: spinach, green beans, broccoli, bok choy, asparagus, seaweed, bell peppers, etc.

In addition to this program, do 20 minutes of sprint intervals 2-3 times per week, separate from your strength training workouts. Don't do steady state cardio, since this will deplete your testosterone and raise your cortisol levels, which will make you lose muscle.

So instead of jogging at the same speed for 30-45 minutes, sprint for as fast and as long as you can (which should be no more than 20 seconds), then walk for 60-90 seconds. Do this repeatedly for about 20 minutes.

And when I mean sprint, I mean an ALL OUT, balls to the wall, full-speed run. If you live in an area with hills, then hill sprints are a good option.

The 6 Factors Program

XVI. The 6 Factors Program

The first 2 volumes of Strength and Physique featured the 6 Factors Program. For an explanation of why the 6 Factors Program works in building muscle, you can read those previous volumes.

For now, understand that the 6 Factors Program is a training template that manipulates the length and intensity of muscular tension to elicit different hormonal and hypertrophic responses. Rather than discuss why the 6 Factors Program works at building muscle, we'll discuss how the program works. In this chapter we'll outline the rules and parameters of this training template.

The 6 Factors Program modulates intensity, volume, density, tension, frequency and variety to elicit and potentiate the anabolic hormones testosterone, growth hormone, insulin, IGF and FGF. Hence, the 6 Factors Program:

- Modulates training volume by alternating between a high number of sets and a low number of sets
- Modulates training intensity by alternating between high reps and low reps
- Modulates time under tension by alternating between extended sets and straight sets
- Modulates training density by alternating between high and low rest periods
- Modulates exercises by varying them throughout the week
- Modulates training frequency by alternating phases of high frequency training and low frequency training

The 6 Factors Program is a training template in which you can plug exercises you feel work best for you. It consists of 4 workouts:

The GH Workouts- These 2 workouts are designed to maximize your output of growth hormone (GH). The workouts do this by utilizing set extenders such as compound sets and trisets. The set extenders increase training density and prolong muscular tension, which leads to increased GH output as well as moderate testosterone output.

GH Workout #1

1. QUADS/HAMSTRINGS triset (2-3 sets, 3-4 minutes rest)
2. CHEST compound set (3-4 sets, 2-3 minutes rest)
3. TRICEPS compound set (4-5 sets, 3-4 minutes rest)

GH Workout #2

1. BACK triset or giant set (3-4 sets, 3-4 minutes rest)
2. DELTOIDS triset (3 sets, 2 minutes rest)
3. BICEPS triset (3 sets, 3 minutes rest)
4. CALVES diminishing sets

The Insulin/Testosterone Sensitizing Workout- This is a full body workout designed to sensitize your body to the anabolic effects of insulin and testosterone. It does this by high employing high reps (insulin sensitization) and high-tension movements (for testosterone receptivity).

Insulin/T Workout

1. CALVES (3 sets, 15-20 reps, 60 seconds rest)
2. DELTOIDS (3 sets, 12-15 reps, 60 seconds rest)
3. CHEST (3 sets, 10-12 reps, 90 seconds rest)
4. BACK (3 sets, 10-12 reps, 90 seconds rest)
5. QUADRICEPS/HAMSTRINGS (3 sets, 10-12 reps, 90 seconds rest)
6. ARMS SUPERSET:
   / BICEPS (3 sets, 12-15 reps, no rest)
   \ TRICEPS (3 sets, 15-20 reps, 90 seconds rest)

The Testosterone Boosting Workout- This also is a full body workout, but it is designed to maximize your body's output of testosterone. It does this by employing heavy compound movements. Heavy compound movements elicit a huge testosterone jolt from your body.

T-Boost Workout

1. CHEST/TRICEPS (4-6 sets, 4-6 reps, 2 minutes rest)
2. BACK/BICEPS (4-6 sets, 4-6 reps, 2 minutes rest)
3. QUADS/HAMSTRINGS (4-6 sets, 4-6 reps, 2 minutes rest)
4. DELTOIDS (4 sets, 10-12 reps, 30 seconds rest)
5. CALVES descending sets (2 series of drop sets, 2 minutes rest)

Cycling through these different workouts throughout the week allows you to gain muscle very quickly. The 6 Factors Microcycle is very tough on the body, however. Your muscles are forced to grow, because the 6 Factors Microcycle is a traumatizing training stimulus. The 6 Factors Program is the SWAT of hypertrophy training: it will hit your muscles with repeatedly brief but overwhelming force.

Hence the 6 Factors Program is recommended only for advanced trainees. Beginning and intermediate trainees should build up their strength and work up to the 6 Factors Program. If you are new to weight training or have been training for less than a year, then you will need to build up the volume and frequency of work before tackling the 6 Factors Microcycle.

The 6 Factors Induction Phase

To ease you into the 6 Factors Program, you can work through an induction phase. This induction phase will slowly introduce to you all the elements of the 6 Factors Program. As you progress through this induction program, you will build up your training frequency. You will cycle from a 2 week high volume phase to a one week low volume phase.

Sunday	Monday	Tuesday	Wednesday	Thursday	Friday	Saturday
	GH #1		GH #2		GH #1	
	GH #2		GH #1		GH #2	
	T-Boost		T-Boost		T-Boost	

You choose what exercises to perform for the GH and T-Boost workouts. Simply plug your favorite exercises into the GH and T-Boost workout templates above and follow the sets, reps and rest periods.

The 6 Factors Microcycle

Once you've completed the 3 week induction phase, you can progress to the 6 Factors Microcycle. The 3 week induction cycle is now compressed into a single week. Cycling your reps within a week is much better, because you will gain size and strength at a faster rate.

For gaining, retaining and building on what you've gained in size, it is always better to train more frequently (3-4 times per week). To train at a high frequency, however, you have to vary the volume from workout to workout. Advanced trainees will need to vary their volume from workout to workout just to keep getting bigger and avoid plateaus. The 6 Factors Microcycle varies the volume build size and muscularity quickly.

Outlined below is the 6 Factors Program. Follow the program as is the first week. Exercise substitutions can be made after you've completed week one. Just make sure to follow the set, rep and rest requirements of the 6 Factors training template.

6 Factors Program

<u>Day 1: GH Workout</u>

Quads Triset:
1. Reverse lunges (5-7 reps)
2. Back squats (perform as many reps as possible with the same weight used for reverse lunges)
3. Sissy squats (as many reps as possible, bodyweight only)
- Perform 3 trisets.
- Rest 3 minutes between trisets.

Chest Compound Set:
1. 20° Dumbbell press (5-7 reps)
2. Pushups (as many reps as possible)
- Perform 2 compound sets.
- Rest 3 minutes between compound sets.

Triceps Compound Set:
1. Lying EZ-bar extensions (5-7 reps)
2. Lying dumbbell extensions (5-7 reps)
- Perform 4 compound sets.
- Rest 4 minutes between compound sets.

<u>Day 2: GH Workout</u>

Back Giant Set:
1. Wide grip pull-ups (as many reps as possible)
2. Medium grip pull-ups (as many reps as possible)
3. Medium grip chin-ups (as many reps as possible)
4. Narrow grip chin-ups (as many reps as possible)
- Perform 3 giant sets.
- Rest 10 seconds between pull-ups. Rest 4 minutes between giant sets.

Deltoid Compound Set:
1. Bradford press (10-12 reps)
2. Wide grip upright rows (perform as many reps as possible with the same weight used in the Bradford press)
- Perform 3 compound sets.
- Rest 2 minutes between compound sets.

Biceps Triset:
1. Incline hammer curls (5-7 reps)
2. Seated dumbbell curls (with the same weight for incline hammer curls perform as many reps as possible)
3. Barbell concentration curls (5-7 reps)
- Perform 3 trisets.
- Rest 3 minutes between trisets.

Calves Diminishing Sets:
- One legged calf raises (100 reps, bodyweight only, alternate between legs with no rest)

Day 3: Off

Day 4: Insulin/T Workout

1) **Standing one legged calf raise** (bodyweight only, 3 sets, as many reps as possible, 60 seconds rest)
2) **Neck press** (3 sets, 10-12 reps, 90 seconds rest)
3) **Elbows out dumbbell rows** (3 sets, 10-12 reps, 90 seconds rest)
4) **One legged squats** (3 sets, as many reps as possible, 90 seconds rest)
5) **Side lying rear flyes** (3 sets, 10-12 reps, 90 seconds rest)
6) Arms Triset:
   a) **Lying dumbbell curls** (6-8 reps)
   b) **Seated dumbbell curls** (as many reps as possible with the same weight used for lying dumbbell curls)
   c) **Diamond pushups** (as many reps as possible)
      o Perform 3 trisets
      o Rest 1 minute between trisets

Day 5: Off

Day 6: T-Boost Workout

1. **Gironda dips** (4 sets, as many reps as possible, 2 minutes rest)
2. **Sternum pull-ups** (4 sets, as many reps as possible, 2 minutes rest)
3. **Deadlifts** (4 sets, 4-6 reps, 2 minutes rest)
4. **Swing lateral raise** (4 sets, 10-12 reps, 30 seconds rest)
5. **Dumbbell calf raises:** 2 series of descending sets (1 set of 8-10 reps followed by 4 drop sets of 8-10 reps each), 2 minutes rest
6. **Arms superset:**
   a) Kettlebell curls (3 sets, 4-6 reps, 90 seconds rest)
   b) One-arm pushups (3 sets, as many reps as possible, 90 seconds rest)

Day 7: Off

Do the 6 Factors Microcycle for 2-3 weeks, and then switch to a different program of your choosing. You can do anything from a powerlifting routine, a bodybuilding routine, a muscle specialization routine or a Crossfit inspired routine.

Most other programs will amp up 1-2 training factors (high volume, heavy weight, etc.), but few will amp up all 6 Factors of hypertrophy. Chances are you will back cycle when you switch from the 6 Factors Program to another program. You will decompress or de-load in some manner: lower training frequency, lower volume, lower density, lower weight, etc.

If you want to extend the life of the 6 Factors Program beyond 3 weeks, then be sure to vary the exercises. You must perform exercises that are completely different from what you've been doing. Even with these changes, you cannot stay on the 6 Factors Program for long. Watch for signs of overtraining:

- Depression
- Loss of strength
- Loss of appetite
- Loss of muscle tone
- Lack of motivation
- Irritability
- Lack of energy

If you experience any of these symptoms and you've been on the 6 Factors Program (or any training program) for longer than 3 weeks, then you will need to back cycle and switch to a decompression program.

You can back cycle from the 6 Factors Program a number of ways:

- **Cut the volume in half**. When in doubt, drop the number of sets to 3 per body part.
- **Decompress the frequency.** Instead of hitting each muscle group 3-4 times a week, drop it down to 1-2 times a week.
- **Abbreviate your exercises.** Stick to one exercise per muscle group, no more.
- **Avoid set extenders and shock techniques.** Just perform straight sets. No trisets, no forced reps, no negatives.

I have found the following types of routines work well as decompression programs following the 6 Factors Microcycle:

1. **Powerlifting programs-** Many powerlifting programs concentrate on just a few exercises (squats, deadlifts and bench press), so these work well as abbreviated workouts.
2. **Prehabilitation programs-** These are programs where you fix any sort of strength imbalances in your body. This could be realigning your posture, strengthening your shoulder joint, strengthening your core or increasing your mobility and flexibility.
3. **Calisthenics-** Doing a bodyweight only workout can serve as a form of active recovery. Performing a calisthenics program for a week or two gives your body a break from heavy lifting. A well-crafted calisthenics program can lubricate the joints and increase mobility and flexibility. Some bodyweight exercises to consider are pushups, pull-ups, chin-ups, dips, bodyweight squats, lunges, hanging leg raises and inverted rows. You should also include some stretching exercises.

Afterword

Atilla the Hun once said, "Superficial goals lead to superficial results."

Likewise, half-ass efforts lead to half-ass results. If you want something badly enough, then you must commit fully and COMPLETELY to doing **everything** to achieve your goal.

This applies especially to physique training and dieting. If you're not willing to diet and exercise, then you should expect a half-ass physique and be happy with it.

But if you're not happy with being average and you want an extraordinary physique, then quit bitching about it and make an extraordinary commitment to doing everything you are supposed to do to get the body you want. No excuses.

Full commitment means hard work and effort, but it also means objectively analyzing what you're doing wrong and what you're doing that's not effective. Don't hold on to misinformation fed to you. If you hold on to the belief that exercising on machines and bouncy blue balls for 15 minutes a day for 2 weeks will get you the warrior physique, then you've been seriously brainwashed by fat-cat marketers. The Greeks and Romans didn't have machines or bouncy balls or fancy equipment. And yet they developed physiques that were literally works of art.

You have to think of training and dieting as a military campaign: it is an all-out assault. Take no prisoners. No compromise. Commit fully, and you will succeed.

Made in the USA
Lexington, KY
28 February 2014